Jill Eckersley is a freelance writer with many years' experience of writing on health topics. She is a regular contributor to women's and general-interest magazines, including *Good Health, Bella, Women's Fitness, Slimming World* and other titles. *Coping with Snoring and Sleep Apnoea, Coping with Childhood Asthma, Coping with Dyspraxia, Coping with Childhood Allergies, Helping Children Cope with Anxiety* and *Every Woman's Guide to Heart Health*, six books written by Jill for Sheldon Press, were all published in 2003–6. She lives beside the Regent's Canal in north London with two cats.

Overcoming Common Problems Series

Selected titles

A full list of titles is available from Sheldon Press,
36 Causton Street, London SW1P 4ST and on our website at
www.sheldonpress.co.uk

Overcoming Common Problems Series

Overcoming Common Problems Series

Overcoming Common Problems

Living with Eczema

JILL ECKERSLEY

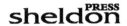

First published in Great Britain in 2007

Sheldon Press
36 Causton Street
London SW1P 4ST

British Library Cataloguing-in-Publication Data
A catalogue record for this book is available from the British Library

ISBN 978-1-84709-011-9

1 3 5 7 9 10 8 6 4 2

Typeset by Fakenham Photosetting Ltd, Fakenham, Norfolk
Printed in Great Britain by Ashford Colour Press

Produced on paper from sustainable forests

Contents

Acknowledgements

I should like to thank the many patient people who have helped me with the research for this book. They include the experts at the National Eczema Society, the British Association of Dermatologists and the British Skin Foundation, especially their ever-helpful press officer, Nina Goad.

Many skin specialists took time out from their busy schedules to talk to me and answer my emails, including Professor Julia Newton Bishop from St James's University Hospital, Leeds, Dr Sue Lewis-Jones from Ninewells Hospital, Dundee, Dr Kim Thomas from Nottingham University, Professor Nick Reynolds from Newcastle University and Professor Irwin McLean from the University of Dundee. Dermatology nurse Moira Craig from Hillingdon Hospital also gave me every assistance, as did the many complementary therapists I spoke to, notably medical herbalist Trudy Norris, doctors Peter Atherton and Ann Williamson, and the staff of the AcuMedic Medical Centre in Camden, London.

Special thanks are due, as always, to the brave souls who talked to me as 'case studies', telling me about their own experience of living with eczema in the hope that their experiences will benefit others. I couldn't have written the book without them. Thank you all.

Acknowledgements

Introduction

Eczema – a condition in which the skin is excessively dry, reddened, often unbearably itchy and inflamed – has become increasingly more common in the UK and other Western countries over the last thirty years. It is now felt that the increase has 'flattened out' over the last decade, at least in the affluent West, although rates are still going up in the developing world. Eczema is related to other allergic conditions like asthma and hay fever, and many people who suffer from one type of allergy find that they are affected by the others as well.

Currently, the National Eczema Society (NES) estimates that as many as *one in twelve* British adults and *one in five* British schoolchildren suffer from eczema. Some children grow out of the condition by the time they go to school, others when they reach puberty. There's still a lot we don't know about eczema, most particularly why there has been such a big increase in the incidence of the condition in recent years. Everything from environmental pollution to our over-clean, poorly ventilated, centrally heated houses and our excessive use of household chemicals has been blamed, but the jury is still out on the causes of eczema, and there is, as yet, no 'cure'. It is not life-threatening – but it *does* affect people's lives, as Diane, 33, explains.

I often think about the life I would have, or could have had, if I didn't have eczema. It affects everything I choose to do and a lot of my choices about what I don't do. It has affected my confidence, as I was bullied as a child because of the state of my skin. Even now, people stare and make comments. It affects the clothes that I wear, the places that I go to, the jobs I apply for, the relationships that I build and the social life that I have – or don't have. It also impacts on big decisions like deciding not to have children.

Diane has extremely severe eczema which affects her whole body from her head right down to her toes. She has tried many forms of treatment, from the conventional to the complementary, and says that what she has found most helpful is accepting that her eczema is with her for life and that she is not one of the lucky ones who will grow out of it.

'I no longer think about the life I can't have; I have learned to live with the condition and to manage it positively,' she says.

Living with eczema, as Diane does, is what this book is about. We shall be looking at healthy skin and its care, as well as investigating what leads so many people to have problem skin. We shall be finding out what those with eczema and their families and friends can do to make living with eczema less of a challenge, whether that means assessing the success of the latest treatments, looking at future research or recommending the lifestyle changes and helpful products which enable those with eczema to lead normal or near-normal lives.

1

Your skin and how to care for it

The skin is the largest organ in the body. It's one which we take for granted until something goes wrong with it. The average adult has about 21 sq ft, or 2 sq m, of skin, weighing 7 lb or 3.2 kg and receiving about one-third of the total blood which is pumped from the heart.

If you looked at your skin under a powerful microscope you would see that it is made up of three layers. The outer layer is called the *epidermis*. It is also divided into layers, the deepest of which is constantly producing new skin cells. The surface of the skin is known as the 'stratum corneum', and consists of dead skin cells filled with keratin – the hard, rigid substance which forms your finger- and toenails. New skin cells eventually work their way up to the surface, where they eventually die and flake off. This is a normal, healthy and continuous process which we don't notice. In fact it has been estimated that the whole skin is replaced about once every four weeks.

Beneath the epidermis is the middle layer of skin, known as the *dermis*. The sebaceous glands in this layer produce lubrication for the surface of the skin in the form of an oily substance called sebum. Sebum acts as a barrier and also a mild antiseptic, although if too much sebum is produced it can block the pores and cause the sort of spots which are the despair of so many teenagers. The dermis contains fibres which give the skin its flexibility, known as 'elastic fibres', and those which give the skin its strength, known as 'collagen fibres'. It also contains sweat glands, hair follicles, connective tissue, white blood cells which help to keep the skin clear of infection, and blood vessels.

Unlike the epidermis, which is practically waterproof, the dermis is permeable, which is why injuries like burns and grazes 'weep' when the tougher epidermis is no longer there to protect them.

The innermost layer of the skin is called the *subcutaneous layer* and consists of fat. This has an insulating effect, rather like a blanket, keeping the cold out when necessary but also allowing heat loss when the body gets very hot. One of the skin's chief and most important functions is to regulate body temperature.

You might also be interested to know that each square half-inch or 1.3 cm of skin contains

- ten hairs;
- 15 sebaceous glands attached to hair follicles;
- 100 sweat glands;
- 1 metre of tiny blood vessels.

The thickness of your skin varies around your body. The palms of your hands and the soles of your feet have the thickest skin, measuring from 1.2 mm to 4.7 mm. This skin is also hair-free or 'glaborous' and produces 'dermatoglyphics' or fingerprints. The thinnest skin is on your lips and eyelids and around your eyes. The skin on most of the body is about 0.6 mm thick and on the face 0.12 mm thick. Babies and elderly people have thinner and more sensitive skin than adults. As we get older we have fewer of the strength-producing collagen fibres in our skin which is why older people's skin tends to wrinkle and sag. (Source: British Association of Dermatologists.)

What is skin for?

Human skin performs several vital functions.

- It protects the inside of your body from injury and environmental damage.
- It acts as a temperature regulator by producing sweat.

- It acts as an immune organ to detect infections.
- It acts as a sensory organ and is vital to your sense of touch, enabling you to tell the difference between heat and cold and recognize pain, itch and vibration.

If the skin fails to perform any of these functions it can lead to health problems. For instance, if the skin stops working as a barrier, the body may lose fluid and become dangerously dehydrated. If it no longer works as a temperature regulator, a person may become a victim of either heat stroke or hypothermia, depending on the temperature. If the skin loses its immune function, the result is an infection, and without the sense of touch there can be problems like bedsores.

The British Association of Dermatologists also point out that the *look* of healthy human skin is very important from a psychological point of view. We expect ordinarily attractive people to have clear, unblemished skin. Anyone with a very dry, cracked, reddened or weeping skin, severe teenage pimples or acne can easily feel that they are being ignored, rejected or ostracized by other people, even though most skin conditions are not contagious. The parents of toddlers with skin conditions notice that, even at nursery, other children sometimes avoid them or don't want to play or hold hands with them. Clear skin is important to our idea of beauty – how many pimply film stars or spotty fashion icons can you name? This has always been so, hence the popularity of so-called 'miracle' creams and face washes designed to give us all perfect skins. Herbal potions and oils, lead pastes and anything from crushed flower petals to petroleum jelly were used in the past; today's women are willing to spend fortunes on little pots of 'scientifically devised' face creams produced by the multi-billion-pound cosmetics industry. In spite of the industry's claims, there seems little evidence that expensive creams work any better than cheaper ones. Research in 2006 from the US Consumer Union and its French counterpart found that the effect of cosmetic preparations on lines and wrinkles was small – less than 10 per cent in most cases – and invisible to the naked eye.

Taking care of your skin

If you really want to take care of your skin, there are plenty of things that you can do to help yourself. Your skin will reflect your general health, and the better you look after yourself – with a healthy diet, plenty of fresh air, sound sleep and regular exercise – the better your skin will look. At the same time, you have to be realistic: no-one can avoid wrinkles for ever and no 60-year-old can expect to have the skin of a 16-year-old. Back in the 1990s, leading neuropsychologist Dr David Weeks studied a group of people he christened the 'Superyoung' – those who looked and acted ten or twenty years younger than their contemporaries. His conclusion was that some skin wrinkles were a result of genetic predisposition but that lifestyle factors like working outdoors in strong sunlight, smoking, diet and poor sleep habits also had an effect on the condition of the skin.

Most skin damage is caused by ultra-violet (UV) light, so the message from skin experts is: stay out of the sun. Between 1975 and 2002, the incidence of skin cancers in British men *quadrupled* and in women rates *tripled*. As well as the much-publicized danger of skin cancer, sunlight causes pigmentation changes, 'liver spots', thinning of the dermis and wrinkles. English women's complexions used to be the envy of the world and were thought to be at least partly the result of our cool, damp climate. Until Coco Chanel made sunbathing fashionable in the 1920s and 1930s, a suntanned appearance was not admired. Ladies in the nineteenth century were careful to shade their pale complexions from blazing sunshine. It's sad if you love sunbathing, but if you bask in the sun like a lizard you risk developing a wrinkled, lizard-like skin. At the very least you should be using a sun cream with a high protection factor.

Smoking is also bad for skin health. In a study of otherwise identical twins carried out by doctors at St Thomas's Hospital in London, the smoking twin looked ten years older than the non-smoker by the age of 40 or so. Think of 'smoked' meat and fish – would you want your complexion looking like that? Smokers' skin can be as much as 40 per cent thinner and more lined than non-smokers'. It seems that some of the harmful chemicals found in cigarette smoke break down collagen, which decreases the natural elasticity of the skin. Smoke also reduces healthy blood flow to the skin and tends to dry out the natural protective oils produced in the dermis.

Changes in the state of your skin can also reflect a deterioration in your general health. Many of us develop spots or dry, rough skin if we are run down or stressed. If you notice your skin becoming much drier than usual, your hair coarsening and your weight increasing, it could be a sign of thyroid problems. Women with severe acne combined with irregular periods and excess hair are sometimes diagnosed with polycystic ovaries.

Do you have dry skin?

Not everyone with dry skin has eczema, but most people with eczema have dry skin. If the skin cells don't contain enough water, then they will shrink and this can lead to tiny cracks appearing in the skin's surface, resulting in a rough appearance and a wrinkled feel. Skin cells which are properly hydrated – containing plenty of water – are healthy and result in the appearance of soft, flexible skin which does its job properly, providing an effective barrier against the environmental factors which could damage it. Dry, cracked skin is much more vulnerable to infection as well.

Apart from conditions such as eczema, there are other reasons why you might have dry skin. Some are unavoidable, such as genetic factors. Dry skin could simply run in your family. The causes of skin problems are complex and seem to involve several different genes rather than just one. Researchers in Dundee in 2006 discovered the gene for dry skin and found that 10 per cent of Europeans were carriers. If one of your parents carries this gene you are likely to have dry skin; if both do, you are at high risk of having eczema. But this is just one piece of the 'eczema jigsaw' and research is ongoing.

It is important for everyone to drink plenty of fluids, and they have to be the right kind of fluids. Water – at least six to eight glasses per day – fruit juices and other non-alcoholic drinks will help to rehydrate your skin as well as flushing out toxins and keeping you healthy in other ways. Drinking more than the recommended amount of alcohol on a regular basis will also dry out your skin, as can excessive coffee consumption. People who have had a fever can also easily become dehydrated as a raised temperature often leads to fluid loss from the body.

Environmental factors can also dry your skin. Living and working in a centrally heated or air-conditioned atmosphere is almost bound to have an effect. We have already mentioned the negative effects of too much sunbathing, but going out on cold, windy days without some protection for your skin can also lead to dry, chapped hands and faces.

Too much washing can dry your skin, especially if you use harsh chemical soaps and detergents. Pollutants you come into contact with at work can lead to skin damage – people like healthcare workers and hairdressers often suffer from skin problems. You may be sensitive to particular substances such as latex (found in rubber gloves), nickel (part of much inexpensive jewellery) or the ingredients in some perfumes and cosmetic products. Most people's skin becomes drier as they get older, though young babies, whose skin hasn't yet developed fully, also suffer from dry skin. Stress can be a factor too.

So what is eczema?

Eczema is more than just dry skin. It is by far the most common problem skin condition, affecting about one in twelve adults and as many as one in five schoolchildren in the country. People with eczema will suffer from some or all of the following symptoms: redness, dryness, flaking skin, skin which cracks and feels painful, unbearable itching, soreness and infection (which is often caused by scratching).

The most common form of eczema, which often runs in families, is called *atopic eczema*. The word 'atopy' refers to the tendency to develop allergic conditions like eczema, but also asthma and hay fever, which are often related. Many (but not all) people who suffer from eczema suffer from other allergic conditions at the same time. In other families, some members have eczema and others one or more of the other allergic conditions. The reason this happens is not known. Atopic eczema usually appears for the first time in childhood – sometimes in babyhood – and about two-thirds of children grow out of the condition.

Eczema is also sometimes known as *dermatitis*, a word which simply means inflammation of the skin. Atopic eczema and atopic dermatitis are the same thing, although 'dermatitis' is more often used to describe the condition which is caused by contact with substances such as chemicals, soap, detergents and even some plants. The National Eczema Society estimates that as many as one in five people will develop some form of dermatitis at some point in their lives after exposure to common household substances such as perfume or hair dye. It's not unusual for people to use a particular product for years with no problems and for eczema to develop quite suddenly and for no apparent reason.

The word 'eczema' comes from ancient Greek and literally means 'to boil over', which is an accurate way of describing how those badly affected by itchy, sore and uncomfortable skin feel.

Eczema can affect any part of the body from the head to the feet, quite literally. Most commonly, it appears in what are known as 'flexural' areas – around the bends of the knees and elbows and around the wrists and neck. You could think of the outer layer of the epidermis – the stratum corneum – as a brick wall, in which the 'bricks' (called corneocytes) are held together by 'cement' (called lipid lamellae). Healthy skin has plenty of cement holding the wall together. The skin of those who have atopic eczema is like an old wall, with the cement cracking and falling away, leaving gaps which allow irritants and allergens to penetrate the skin, causing the soreness and itching eczema sufferers know only too well.

Other forms of eczema

There are other kinds of eczema in addition to atopic eczema. *Contact dermatitis* is caused by the skin coming into contact with substances which irritate it and cause a reaction. There are two kinds of contact dermatitis, although as the symptoms are very similar (dry, reddened, cracked, sore or weeping skin, with or without skin burns, ulcers and fluid-filled blisters) it can be difficult to tell them apart without 'patch testing' (see p. 74). In cases of *irritant contact dermatitis*, the skin problems develop when there has been direct contact with damaging or irritating substances. Many workers whose hands are in water a lot or who are in occupations which bring them into contact with chemicals in one form or another – for example, hairdressers, nurses, caterers, cleaners, metalworkers and construction workers – are often affected by irritant contact dermatitis, which can lead to time off work and loss of earnings. *Allergic contact dermatitis* produces many of the same symptoms, but is the result of an allergic reaction which can be identified by allergy testing (see p. 18).

Seborrhoeic eczema is better known as 'cradle cap' when it appears in babies. Cradle cap leads to a greasy, scaly scalp and sometimes scaly or roughened patches on other parts of the baby's body. It looks unattractive but generally does not bother the baby very much and often clears up of its own accord without any treatment. In older people, seborrhoeic eczema also starts on the scalp, with severe, greasy dandruff being one of the first symptoms. The scalp becomes extremely itchy and the skin sore and sensitive, with a rash affecting the 'greasier' parts of the skin, for example parts of the face and the edges of the scalp. The area behind the ears is often affected and this can lead to irritation inside the ear. Other parts of the body can also be affected.

According to the latest research from the National Eczema Society, the cause of seborrhoeic eczema is still unclear, although a yeast called *pityrosporum ovale* has been found on the skin of people with this condition and this may form part of the cause.

There is also *pompholyx eczema*, where uncomfortable blisters appear on the fingers, hands and feet, and *discoid eczema*, which leads to coin-shaped patches on the arms and legs. In both these types of eczema there is a risk of the skin blistering and drying out, allowing skin infections to develop.

Gravitational eczema affects the lower legs and is associated with high blood pressure in the veins in that part of the body. Deep vein thrombosis, phlebitis and varicose veins can also lead to this type of eczema, in which the skin around the ankles and lower legs becomes thin, blistered, shiny and cracked. Leg ulcers which are difficult to heal can be a complication of this form of eczema.

Sometimes eczema is made worse by exposure to the sun's UV rays, even on cloudy days. Elderly people whose skin has stopped producing enough protective sebum can develop particularly eczema-like dry skin conditions.

Sore, broken and damaged skin is particularly vulnerable to bacterial infections, most of which can be treated with antibiotics.

A more serious complication can arise if someone with atopic eczema becomes infected with the *herpes simplex* or cold sore virus, leading to a condition called *eczema herpeticum*. Small groups of fluid-filled blisters can appear anywhere on the body, and in severe cases the person develops a high temperature and feels generally unwell. Should this happen you are advised to contact your GP as drug treatments are available.

The effects of eczema

Eczema is not life-threatening and it is not contagious, but at present there is no cure and the management of the condition can involve lifestyle changes, not only for the one with eczema but also for his or her family. There are medical treatments such as emollient creams and steroids (see Chapter 5). Complementary therapies ranging from herbal potions and traditional Chinese medicine to Dead Sea mud and treatment with alpine spa water (see Chapter 8) seem to work for some people. Those living with eczema have to get used to avoiding the 'triggers' for their skin condition, which can be anything from animal hair to washing powder, and have to adjust their lives accordingly. Living with sore, itchy, painful skin can affect your life in so many ways, from your self-confidence to your sleep patterns, as Diane explains.

> The state of my skin will generally affect my mood for the day. If I have to spend it wearing bandages or a full body suit, I will feel heavy and constrained by the bandages, but I will also not be scratching, as it's usually too much of an effort to take them off! I have to take spare clothes with me to work in case I have a reaction. I have tubs of moisturizing cream with me in my office to help keep my skin moist and I also drink a lot of water to achieve the same.
>
> I am careful about the environments I go into. Even in shops I have to stay away from the perfume counters. If my skin is really bad I have to stay away from the gym as getting hot and sweaty when I exercise makes the eczema sting more. When I am hot, itchy or sore,

getting to sleep is a nightmare and I will, on occasion, scratch myself until I bleed.

The National Eczema Society says that the effects of eczema are often underestimated. The itching and soreness can cause great distress, and some people with eczema feel that they are so disfigured by it that they are reluctant to go out or mix with others at social events and especially to wear skin-revealing clothes or swimming costumes. If not properly managed, eczema can prevent children going to school and cause people to leave their jobs. There is, at present, no cure for eczema. Although many children grow out of it, some have to live with it in adult life too. The purpose of this book is to show how the condition can be treated and 'managed' so that those with eczema can lead a normal or near-normal life.

2

What can go wrong

It is known that eczema, like other allergic conditions, has become much more common in today's world. What is not known is exactly why this should be, although there are lots of theories. There seems to be something about the way we live in the developed world in the twenty-first century which has led to 'atopy' (the tendency to develop allergic conditions like eczema) becoming far more widespread. There are far more cases of eczema and other allergic conditions in affluent Western societies than there are in the developing world, and no-one as yet has discovered the reason. Research is helping to build up a picture of the allergy jigsaw, but not nearly enough is known to make the picture a complete one yet.

Outdoor air pollution, including the huge rise in the numbers of cars on the roads producing high levels of sulphur dioxide, carbon monoxide, nitrogen dioxide and ozone, could be a factor. The *type* of air pollution could make a difference, since fifty years ago the air in the UK's towns and cities was polluted by coal fires and the fumes from factory chimneys. In one notorious episode of 'smog' or polluted fog in 1950s London, around 4,000 people died. After the fall of the Berlin Wall in 1989, researchers found out that the incidence of allergies in the heavily industrialized East had actually been lower than in the West, but in about five years the former East Germans had caught up. In the UK, because of the prevailing winds, it's hard to say whether 'country' air is actually cleaner than city air. High levels of ozone have been recorded in Somerset, rural Oxfordshire and the Sussex coast. At the moment, there seems to be no *direct* correlation between air pollution and eczema or other allergic conditions, although there does seem to be slightly more eczema in busy urban areas than in the countryside. A research study in 2000 found that the highest rates of eczema in the UK seemed to be in the north Midlands, eastern England, London and southern and south-east England. Curiously, these were not the areas where other allergic conditions like asthma and hay fever were most common.

Could indoor air pollution be a factor? We use an increasing number of chemicals in our everyday lives for everything from fireproofing our furniture to colouring our hair or cleaning our bathrooms. Our well-insulated and centrally heated modern homes are ideal breeding-grounds for house-dust mites, which can trigger off an eczema flare-up in some people. It has even been suggested that one of the reasons why eczema affects so many of today's children is because they are the victims of our 'indoor' culture, spending too much time playing computer games or watching TV rather than playing outdoors in the fresh air. However, it is worth remembering that Australia and New Zealand, countries with generally healthy outdoor lifestyles, have even higher rates of allergic disease than the UK does.

There is also the 'Hygiene Hypothesis', suggested as long ago as 1989 by an epidemiologist called David Strachan, which states that we all live in such clean homes these days that our bodies are vulnerable to all sorts of conditions which would not have been a problem in the past. It is known that people growing up on farms, who are exposed to animal dander (a combination of hair and saliva) and farmyard muck from an early age, are less likely to develop allergies. We certainly wash both ourselves and our clothes, often using detergent-based soaps and bath preparations and chemical-based detergents, far more frequently than was the case fifty years ago. This could contribute to the increase in the amount of eczema, with the skin's protective natural oils simply being washed away.

Another theory mentions the ' Idling Immune System'. This suggests that cells in our bodies that once would have developed as the TH–1 types, which fight off infectious diseases, are now developing as TH–2 cells, which seem to cause allergy problems, now that once-common infectious diseases are so much less of a threat to our health. This could explain why there are fewer allergies in the developing world, where infectious diseases are still common – although allergies are on the rise in the developing world too.

However, there doesn't seem to be any *single* reason why so many of us are developing allergies, including eczema, and for that reason it is acknowledged as a 'multi-factorial' condition. As far as is known, the causes of eczema seem to be a combination of *genetic* and *environmental* factors. Eczema is not particularly common in the hot, humid air of the tropics, but when, for example, Pakistani or Bangladeshi families come to live in cold, chilly Britain, their children are much more likely to develop it.

In practical terms, what this tends to mean is that it's only by trial and error that people with eczema find out what causes their own particular flare-ups, and discover what kind of treatment helps them to deal with the flare-ups when they happen. Heat, stress, house-dust mites and pet dander are among the 'triggers' for some people's eczema, but every case is different. This means that finding the best way to manage your eczema can sometimes be a slow and frustrating process.

What is atopy?

We have already learned that atopy is the tendency to develop an allergic condition like eczema and that it is often inherited. But what does that actually mean?

To understand atopy, you need to understand how the body's immune system works. Our immune systems are designed to react to genuine 'attackers' such as viruses and bacteria, by producing antibodies to fight them off. People with atopic conditions basically have over-active immune systems which react to substances or conditions that, in non-atopic people, wouldn't cause any problems. In other words, if your eczema flares up when you wear a woolly jumper or use a chemical cleaning product or hair dye, it means that your immune system perceives this as a threat and starts to defend itself by producing antibodies to attack the ' dangerous' substance.

The allergy antibody is called Immunoglobulin E or IgE. Non-atopic people usually have only small amounts of IgE in their systems. If you are atopic, your immune system starts to produce a large amount of the IgE antibody when it detects a substance which would be harmless in unaffected people. This leads to a complex chain of events in your body and ultimately to the symptoms typical of an allergic reaction – swelling, redness, soreness and itching. It is not yet known why some people in atopic families develop eczema, others asthma or hay fever and others none of these.

What's the difference between atopic eczema and the other kinds of eczema?

Non-atopic eczema develops as a result of contact with a substance which does not lead to an allergic response. In other words, your body does not produce IgE antibodies, and the common allergy tests such as skin-prick or blood tests have a negative result.

Can eczema be prevented?

If you know you have allergies in the family – if you and/or your partner suffer or suffered as children from any of the allergic conditions – you might wonder if there is anything you can do to avoid passing on eczema to your children. The short answer is: not a lot. Research has been done to find out whether what mums do or don't do during pregnancy makes a difference to their babies' eczema, but results are not conclusive. A study reported in the *British Journal of Dermatology* in 2001 found that there was a stronger link between mothers' allergies and their babies' eczema than there was for fathers' allergies, and that babies born to more highly educated mothers with smaller families were more likely to have eczema. Some mothers with allergies in the family say they tried to avoid known allergens like peanuts during their pregnancy, or that avoiding cow's milk when they were breast-feeding seemed to improve their babies' skin condition, but there don't seem to be any hard and fast rules. For more detailed information about how diet, especially during pregnancy, can affect babies, see Chapter 7.

3

Eczema in children and teenagers

Childhood eczema is extremely common, with the National Eczema Society estimating that as many as one in five children might be affected to some degree. That means that in an average school class of 30 children, six may have eczema. The condition can affect children psychologically, as well as physically, and can make life difficult in all sorts of ways. Some children's eczema is very obvious, so that they are bullied or teased for looking 'different'. Eczema flare-ups can be triggered by all sorts of things from heat to synthetic clothing to food, so sunny classrooms, nylon sports gear and anything from the class hamster or guinea-pig to the chemicals used in a science class can cause a reaction.

Not all the difficulties caused by living with eczema are that obvious. Sleep problems, both for children with eczema and for their parents, are a common side-effect. Children who are kept awake at night by sore, bleeding and uncomfortable skin can fall behind with their school work or seem lazy and inattentive in class. They may need to take more time off than other children for hospital appointments, leading to accusations of skiving.

Teenagers may have particular problems. At an age when they are beginning to worry about looking good, being in with the in crowd or attracting the opposite sex, it isn't easy to deal with red, itchy, angry skin. At a time when they want to make a life for themselves and become increasingly independent, family relationships can be difficult if Mum is still 'fussing' about using protective emollients and staying out of the sun. Even their choice of career options can be limited if they have severe eczema, with a question mark over careers like hairdressing, the police and Armed Forces, or healthcare jobs. Stress can cause eczema flare-ups and these might, for unlucky teens, coincide with examination times. A Scottish study of 379 young people between the ages of 5 and 16 and their parents, published in 2006 in the *British Journal of Dermatology*, found that severe eczema and other serious skin conditions affected the youngsters' quality of life to the same extent as other chronic diseases such as epilepsy, diabetes or kidney disease. Just because eczema isn't life-threatening, it doesn't mean it's easy to live with, as parents of young people with eczema soon discover.

Some children are only mildly affected and their parents find that, with careful management, eczema is no more than a nuisance. Jenny, mother of five-year-old Ben, says exactly that.

> I have very dry skin myself but as far as I know there are no other allergies in my family or my husband's. When Ben was born with red patches around his wrists and ankles and under his arms, I didn't really know what it was. Ben was quite a miserable baby who cried a lot, and it was easy to see how uncomfortable his skin was.
>
> I asked the nurses at the baby clinic what they thought the problem was. They said it looked like eczema and recommended that I tried various over-the-counter creams and bath products which they said might help. I experimented a bit and ended up putting Oilatum in his bath, which helped a lot. I'd always used a lot of baby lotion and creams but I switched to E45 cream, and that seemed to work. I can't say it's very user-friendly as it is rather thick and I have to wait till it dries on his skin before dressing him, but it is very effective.
>
> We've been lucky compared with some children. With the help of his creams and moisturizers, Ben's skin seems to be all right though it does flare up occasionally. I'm careful to dress him in cotton clothes and keep him out of the sun, but basically it's a question of keeping his skin moisturized.
>
> As he's got older I've learned he is allergic to eggs and his skin flares up if he comes into contact with some dogs, but that's all. He's not self-conscious about his skin and we haven't run into any problems at nursery or school.

At the other end of the spectrum is Sian's son Simon, now seven, whose eczema was extremely severe. Fortunately there was a specialist allergy unit attached to Sian's local hospital so Simon was able to obtain very effective treatment.

> My message would be that you don't have to wait until your child grows out of it. Simon's skin erupted – that isn't too strong a word – when he was eight weeks old. I had no experience of anything like it. There's asthma in my husband's family but that's all.
>
> Simon was literally tortured by his skin. The eczema covered him from head to toe, poor little mite, even his eyes and his eyelids. He looked so awful I was ashamed, I thought everyone must think we were dirty or something. It was obvious he was hurting; he would wriggle when we held him and scratch himself until his skin bled. We hardly got any sleep and we were at our wits' end worrying about him.
>
> My health visitor was very kind and made sure we got our referral to the allergy unit, who couldn't have been more helpful. A consultant assessed Simon and told us that although he might very well grow out of it there was no reason why we should all suffer until he did!

Sian and her husband were introduced to the technique of 'wet-wrapping' their small son, which involved bathing him in emollient and then applying hydrocortisone ointment all over his body before wrapping him in a layer of damp bandages, and then another layer of dry bandages. The bandages had to be changed twice a day, and although it was extremely time-consuming and difficult at first, Sian found that it transformed the family's lives immediately.

> It was like a miracle. He started to sleep properly and that gave us our first chance since his birth to sleep as well. The morning after his first wet-wrapped night, he actually laughed for the first time ever.
>
> The allergy clinic took a multi-faceted approach to Simon's care, giving him RAST tests to establish any allergies and replacing his top-up formula feeds with a special hypo-allergenic formula called Nutramigen.
>
> The tests seemed to be very accurate. We were told he was moderately allergic to cow's milk and other things like eggs, fish and corn. When it came to weaning him, some of these items seemed to upset his tummy if I tried to give them to him, but it only seemed to be milk that caused the eczema to flare up. We changed his diet and used the emollients we had been given and gradually we found we had to wet-wrap

him less and less often as his skin calmed down. By the time he was a year old he only had a couple of little patches behind his knees and on his arms.

Prevention is better ...

Since many – though by no means all – cases of eczema and other allergic conditions run in families, parents often wonder if there is anything they can do to make it less likely their child will be born with a difficult skin.

As it is not yet known exactly why children develop *particular* allergies – in atopic families some children get asthma, others eczema, others hay fever, a combination of all these or nothing at all – it isn't easy to suggest helpful strategies for parents-to-be. Some experts suggest that mums-to-be should try to minimize their exposure to known allergens like house-dust mite and pet dander during pregnancy, and avoid eating peanuts or peanut products. Pregnant women need a healthy diet containing foods from all the major food groups. For the latest information on healthy eating in pregnancy, contact the Sainsbury's/WellBeing Helpline (for contact details see Useful addresses). It is also recommended that you breast-feed your baby for six months, as breast-feeding does help to confer immunity. However, it is not known whether what you eat (or avoid eating) while you are breast-feeding will make any difference, and research into the subject has produced inconclusive results.

Caring for a baby with eczema

Moisturizers and emollients, which come in the form of bath products, lotions, creams and ointments, are the first line of defence if your baby has eczema. Dermatologists recommend asking the advice of your health visitor or GP and starting treatment with emollients as soon as you notice your baby's skin is affected, rather than letting the condition get worse.

Most 'ordinary' baby products, however mild and gentle, contain chemicals which can cause an allergic reaction. There are some specially formulated organic ranges such as those by Green People and Jurlique (for contact details see Useful addresses) which can be suitable for babies with very sensitive skins. Some of the smaller companies were actually founded by people who couldn't find any products suitable for their eczema-affected children. A word of caution, however. Just because a baby product is labelled organic or is plant-based it doesn't always mean it won't cause a reaction in your baby. Trial and error is the best way to find emollients which suit your child. Many can be bought over the counter. Ask your pharmacist's advice on which are suitable for babies and small children. Names to look out for include Oilatum, the E45 range and the Dermol range. Both E45 and Oilatum produce a special children's range of products which are widely available. You can replace ordinary baby wipes with damp cotton wool or kitchen towel moisturized with emollient, and wash your baby's hair in bath water containing emollient bath oil.

There are also companies that make special clothing for babies and children with skin problems (for details see Useful addresses). Synthetic fabrics are best avoided; most parents find that pure cotton or silk suits their children best. Many outfits are made with the seams and labels on the outside to avoid rubbing against sore skin. It's important to keep the baby's fingernails cut short so she can't scratch. Soft mittens are also available, as are special sleepsuits with attached mittens. The National Eczema Society can advise you on suitable clothing ranges and also on allergy-proof bedding.

We shall be looking at lifestyle changes you can make in Chapter 6. There is still some disagreement about exactly how necessary – and effective – it is to do things like getting rid of carpets and upholstered furniture, but many parents say they are willing to try anything that might help, especially when there are reasonably priced alternatives, like leather or cane furniture, wood or laminate floors, and blinds to replace heavy curtains which attract dust.

Heat also seems to affect many children with eczema; it's suggested that you keep your home at a temperature around 18 degrees C. Very hot baths and showers should also be avoided as hot water can dry out and irritate sensitive skin.

Soft toys can be put in plastic bags and left in the freezer overnight to kill any house-dust mites.

Vaccinations

Some people seem to be afraid that vaccinating their children against the most common childhood diseases may lead to a flare-up of their eczema but the British Association of Dermatologists has found no links between vaccination and eczema in children.

Children and steroids

We shall be looking at the use of corticosteroids, to give steroids their full name, in more detail in Chapter 5. They are potent drugs and many parents are understandably concerned about giving them to children, even when they are prescribed by doctors. Part of the problem is that they are confused with the anabolic steroids used illegally by some athletes and bodybuilders, though they are not the same drugs.

Steroids prescribed to treat skin conditions like eczema are related to the hormones naturally produced by human adrenal glands. Creams and ointments containing steroids are given to relieve the itching and inflammation caused by eczema when treatment with emollients alone does not seem to offer relief. Steroid treatment can be extremely effective, even for babies. Steroids vary in potency, with hydrocortisone being the mildest.

Doctors normally prescribe the lowest effective potency of a particular steroid, and since the vast majority of children with eczema need only intermittent steroid treatment in addition to their usual emollients, there is no reason why steroids cannot be used.

Steroids have been used to treat childhood eczema for thirty years or more and have a good general safety record. Like all drugs, they can have side-effects – notably thinning of the skin – and may not suit everyone. Your child may be prescribed a more potent steroid for use on some areas of the body, for instance arms and legs, and a milder version for facial use. It's important to make sure you know exactly how and for how long to use the steroid cream you have been prescribed.

Eczema at nursery and school

It isn't, of course, parents alone who need to know how to care for children with eczema. Grandparents, childminders, nannies and nursery-school teachers will all need to be made aware of your child's special needs. Fortunately, in a sense, eczema and other allergies are now so common that most nurseries and schools are reasonably familiar with the care that must be taken.

Even so, they don't know *your* child, so before she starts nursery or school it's always advisable to have a chat with her carers and explain what needs to be done for her. It could be something as simple as supplying a soft cotton towel of her own and some emollient, so that any itching or soreness can be dealt with on the spot, or making sure she is able to sit in the shade so that bright sunshine doesn't cause a flare-up. Discuss with your child's carer or teacher

- the kind of treatment she needs and how time-consuming it is likely to be;
- whether she will need time off school for hospital appointments and so on;

- whether sleep problems are likely to mean she gets especially tired and needs more 'quiet time' than other children;
- which activities may possibly cause problems, for example painting and craft work, sand-and-water play or contact with pets;
- if her eczema is known to be diet-related, what she can and can't eat.

The National Eczema Society has a 'Schools Pack' with appropriate information for both parents and teachers. Clearly the situation will change as your child gets older, and especially as eczema tends to 'come and go', but the basic care involved remains the same.

Older children will need to be taught to use their own emollient and it's important to stress that clean hands are vital! It can be helpful to decant a small amount of your child's medication into a discreet little pot which is easy to carry in a schoolbag. By the time your child is in primary school you will probably be aware of the trigger factors for her eczema. These may affect some of her classroom activities and even her school uniform if her skin is sensitive to synthetics. There are companies which supply pure cotton school clothing and protective cotton gloves which could enable her to take part in painting or science classes. See 'Useful addresses' for details.

There are ways round most of the practical problems your child might face in school. Cotton gloves can be worn for art, craft or food technology classes. Extremes of temperature can be avoided. Cotton sportswear can be worn. Don't let your child's eczema stop her living a normal, healthy life!

Stress can exacerbate eczema in children and teenagers and this can have an effect on exam results. If this is a problem for your child you'll need to ensure that the school knows about it. Examination boards are sympathetic to young people whose performance may be affected by medical conditions (hay fever is often at its worst during the exam season). Talk this possibility over with your child's teacher and take the appropriate steps to let the examination board know in plenty of time if there is likely to be a problem.

It's natural to worry when you hand over your child to the care of others but it's important that she feels confident about being able to manage her eczema. The more confident she feels, the less she is likely to be troubled by any stares or comments from the other children. It can't be stated too often that eczema is *not* catching and has *nothing* to do with personal hygiene. A well-adjusted child will be able to tell her friends that she has a 'tickly skin' and needs to put 'special cream' on it to stop it getting sore.

Sadly, children who are, or look, 'different' can sometimes be bullied or picked on by others and we all know how cruel children and young people can be. These days schools are much more aware of bullying than they used to be and are supposed to have policies in place to deal with it if it does occur. The days when the misery and fear it caused were regarded with complacency as 'just part of growing up' are, thankfully, behind us. If you suspect that your child is being bullied because of eczema, reassure the child and then contact the school to find out what steps they can take to resolve the issue. Both ChildLine and Kidscape (for contact details see Useful addresses) have made special studies of bullying and can offer all kinds of strategies to help young people cope.

Eczema and teenagers

Many parents feel that teenagers have quite enough to cope with today, what with exams and career choices, and pressures to be 'cool' and have the latest fashions and gadgets, to be in with the in crowd and to look good and attract the opposite sex. Growing up is not easy for any teen, without the added pressure caused by an unpredictable and uncomfortable condition like eczema. It's also disappointing if you (and your child) have been told that he or she is likely to grow out of it, and then this doesn't happen. It is known that young people with any kind of chronic health condition are more likely to suffer from emotional disturbance than those without, but it's not a simple equation.

Whether your child finds the teenage years a breeze or a roller-coaster ride of moods and difficulties depends on so many things. Family relationships, his own personality and the circumstances he finds himself in can all play a part. What can a caring parent do to help?

The National Eczema Society has special leaflets aimed at teens, with a lot of helpful tips and hints plus quotes from other teenagers dealing with the same issues. However self-conscious teens are about their appearance, they need to be reminded that *nobody*'s perfect. All those gorgeous models and movie stars whose photos appear in magazines and on TV have armies of stylists and make-up artists behind them, not to mention all the computer trickery that can airbrush out any skin blemishes and transform a star's appearance. If your daughter's skin isn't her best feature, there will be something else which is – beautiful eyes, good legs, silky hair, an appealing laugh. These days young men as well as young women are encouraged to take care of themselves and their health and well-being, as well as their looks.

When it comes to making friends and attracting the opposite sex, a warm, friendly personality, a good sense of humour and a genuine interest in other people are what matter. Plus, good grooming. Even though many of the lotions and potions on the chemist's shelves are unsuitable for sensitive skins, it's vital – and simple – for teens and their clothes to be clean and fresh. Many companies do produce hypo-allergenic cosmetics and toiletries (see information in Useful addresses).

Letting go

Perhaps the most useful thing that any parent of a teenager with eczema can do is arm them with the sort of self-confidence and self-esteem to face any problems their condition may lead to. The National Eczema Society's leaflets for teens are helpful. If your teen is seeing a specialist it can also help to let her talk to the consultant alone, to ask any questions for herself and find out as much as she can about the everyday realities of living with her condition. Being well-informed and matter-of-fact about eczema and what it means can also be useful if she is teased or questioned by friends and schoolmates.

It is also worth remembering as GCSE choices approach that severe eczema can affect career choices. Any job that brings a person into contact with chemicals or where a lot of hand-washing is required can cause difficulties for those whose eczema is likely to flare up. Hairdressing, kitchen work, animal handling and car mechanics are among the careers which might pose problems. In cases of very severe eczema which seems to be triggered by the environment, even having to work in a dusty office or a very dry air-conditioned environment can cause difficulties. The National Eczema Society has a factsheet, 'Working with Eczema', which has a lot of helpful tips.

Kick Asthma Holidays, run by Asthma UK and aimed at children and young people between the ages of 6 and 17, welcome youngsters with eczema and other allergic conditions as well as asthma. In addition to normal holiday activities like sports and visits to theme parks, the holidays include information about living with allergies and provide the chance to meet other youngsters with the same problems (see Useful addresses for contact details).

4

Eczema day to day

It's like having thousands of little insects crawling under your skin – at home, at work, when I'm out trying to enjoy myself, all the time. People who don't have eczema can't imagine what it's like unless you tell them to remember having a really itchy insect bite that they were desperate to scratch. Well, that's what it's like for people like me. Except that my skin doesn't heal, or stop itching. Ever.

It wasn't unusual for me to have to get up to my son 14 times a night to change his dressings, which would become soaked with blood as he scratched himself. He couldn't sleep, and cried, and my husband and I didn't get much rest either.

If you ask most people with eczema what is the worst thing about their condition, they will tell you it's the itch – that maddening feeling that makes them desperate to obtain the relief that comes with scratching. Except that scratching brings only a temporary respite from the itching. Scratching is what raises red weals and rashes on sensitive skin, and the more you dig your nails in, the greater the risk of broken, bleeding skin ... which in its turn is much more vulnerable to infection, and more soreness and itching.

If your skin is particularly itchy in one area the temptation is to go on and on scratching there, which leads to a process called lichenification. This is where the skin starts to thicken and even change colour, giving the patches a leathery appearance and contrasting with the areas of unaffected skin. Without treatment and proper management, the more your skin itches, the more you scratch, and the more it itches. This is known as the 'itch–scratch cycle'. Controlling eczema means somehow managing to break this cycle so that your skin has a chance to heal.

Why does your skin itch?

As yet, researchers have not discovered the answer to this question. Skin which is affected by eczema releases chemicals which stimulate the nerves, which in their turn pass the 'itch' sensation to the brain. It used to be thought that *histamine* was one of the chief chemicals causing this, and anti-histamines were prescribed by doctors to treat itching. More recent research has found that histamine may not be the most important chemical involved, although anti-histamines are still sometimes prescribed. Their sedative effect may help people sleep who would otherwise be kept awake by itching.

Everyone who has eczema needs to learn to recognize his or her own 'triggers' – the situations or substances which will make the eczema flare up in the first place, and which make an itch worse. Triggers are different for everyone but among the most common ones are heat, sweating, particular fabrics (both clothing and bedding), environmental factors like house-dust mites or pet dander, common chemicals such as those found in soap, detergents, make-up and household products, pollens, even some foods. Some unlucky people find that almost anything can start off the itch–scratch cycle, as Diane explains.

I have been patch tested and given a four-page list of triggers, so it's easier to say what doesn't affect me rather than what does! Animal hair, especially dogs, synthetic materials, washing powders, soaps, make-up, other people's perfume, scented products including cleaning fluids, central heating, cigarette smoke and stress are among the most usual.

I have to be careful whose house I go to because of dust and animal dander, and it has been difficult to find a job that doesn't aggravate my skin condition. I can't go to a club and dance the night away with my friends because the combination of smoke, heat and sweat will set my eczema raging. Or rather, I can do things, but I always have to think of the consequences.

'Patch testing' (see p. 74) can sometimes be helpful in identifying triggers, but it is not always 100 per cent reliable and many people find that trial and error is the best way for them to find out what is most troublesome, starting with the most common triggers:

- Heat and temperature generally: many people find that a change in temperature, for instance when they get dressed or undressed, is enough to start off an itch. Overheating in bed at night is a common cause of problems.
- Sweating: sweat can irritate sore skin. Sportspeople and gym-goers may find that the hotter and sweatier they get, the worse their eczema becomes.
- Unsuitable clothing: many people, not just those with eczema, find that they can't wear wool next to their skin. Synthetic fibres such as Lycra can also cause problems. Bulky and rough seams can rub and irritate sore, reddened or flaking skin.
- Allergens: allergens like pollen – from trees, grasses or mould spores – can set up all kinds of reactions including eczema. House-dust mites, tiny creatures which live in the carpets, upholstery and bedding of even the cleanest homes, can also set up a reaction. All kinds of household chemicals, flowers and plants, pets and some kinds of foodstuffs can cause a flare-up in susceptible people. One research study found that the average woman uses at least 12 toiletry products every day, containing up to 175 different chemicals which may irritate sensitive skin.
- Stress: many people find that stressful situations make their eczema worse. This can be another vicious circle as worrying about the state of your skin can be stressful in itself. (See the section on stress on pp. 63–8.)

Coping with itching

The first step is to avoid as many of your known triggers as you can. This isn't always easy, of course, and can be quite impossible unless you are able to live in a sterile bubble. Even if you and your family don't use any perfume or household chemicals and manage to find alternatives which suit you, life can be difficult if you have to avoid carpeted offices, plants and flowers in the home or staffroom, even the perfume counter in your local department store. Some very sensitive people flare up if, for instance, they come into contact with someone who owns a cat or dog, and you can't always avoid pet-owning friends and family.

Always keep your skin well moisturized. We shall be looking at *emollients*, the range of lotions, creams and ointments you can buy from pharmacists or be prescribed by your doctor, in detail in Chapter 5. Whatever emollient you use, don't be afraid to use plenty of it so that your sensitive skin does not get a chance to dry out. As we have said, dry, cracked skin is much more vulnerable to bacterial infection and also to the irritation caused by contact with chemicals and other allergens. Don't rub your emollient in: smooth it on gently, as rubbing too hard can make the itching worse.

Make sure your nails are kept short and neatly trimmed so that if you do succumb to scratching there is less change of damaging delicate skin. It is often suggested that children with eczema wear cotton mittens in bed. If scratching at night is a problem for you as an adult, you can do the same.

Don't have your bath or shower too hot, use a suitable emollient bath oil, and pat yourself dry with a soft towel. Don't scrub or rub your skin.

Try to take your mind off the itch by doing something else – reading, watching a DVD, working, chatting – anything! The National Eczema Society suggests you clench your fists tightly when you feel the urge to scratch and hold them clenched for 30 seconds, during which time you could try to divert your attention away from the itch.

If you have to touch your skin, stroking or pinching might be less damaging and destructive than scratching it. Some people find something cool is soothing – such as ice cubes wrapped in a clean cotton tea towel.

Wear several thin layers of suitable (cotton or silk) clothing so that you never get too hot and can adjust your body temperature as often as necessary.

Sleep problems

Sleep problems are extremely common among those with eczema and their families. All parents know how draining it can be to care for a sleepless baby or toddler, and someone whose skin is constantly itching is almost bound to have difficulty falling and staying asleep. Sleep deprivation can actually be quite dangerous in the long term, leading to exhaustion, irritability, poor concentration at school or work, and falling asleep at inappropriate times, all of which can affect family relationships.

People need varying amounts of sleep but we all need to go through a number of 'sleep cycles' consisting of lighter, dreaming and non-dreaming, and very deep restorative sleep. Anyone, child or adult, who persistently misses out on sleep is bound to find that it affects their physical, mental and emotional health. According to the National Eczema Society, studies show that children with atopic eczema spent between 13 and 136 minutes each night scratching, and scratched between 20 and 97 times per night. It's clear that these children are going to have very disturbed sleep patterns, and so are the adults who care for them.

You can improve your chances of a good night's sleep by having a regular, soothing bedtime routine consisting of a warm bath, perhaps a milky drink, a bit of undemanding reading or a TV programme – or a bedtime story if the person with eczema is a child. Relaxation therapies (see pp. 91–5) and products like anti-allergy bedlinen (see Useful addresses) can also be helpful. It's advisable to keep your bedroom comfortably cool, with the windows open and the central heating off or at a very low temperature. Several thin layers of blankets are better than a thick, heavy duvet. Vacuuming the mattress regularly may help, especially if you use a vacuum cleaner with an HEPA (high-efficiency particulate air) filter, which is specially designed to filter out dust-mite particles and pollen. Twin beds may enable someone with eczema and his or her partner to get a better night's sleep. Although it can be tempting for parents to take their sleepless baby or toddler into bed with them, when eczema is the problem this can often make matters worse as the increased body heat just increases the itching.

If you are suffering from sleepless nights in spite of home remedies and relaxation, don't be afraid to go back to your GP for help. Sleep problems are incredibly common and help is available – not all of it in the form of 'sleeping pills'. Yoga, autogenic training, hypnotherapy and other techniques can be extremely useful, and there are also specialized sleep clinics at some hospitals. Ask your GP if you think this might be helpful for you.

The psychological impact of eczema

It isn't just their physical discomfort which people with eczema find so distressing. Eczema is a very visible condition and this can cause psychological problems for both children and adults. According to NES surveys, 86 per cent of those with the condition say they feel self-conscious about their skin and 88 per cent say that stress can trigger their eczema or make it worse.
As Sue, 23, says:

> I know people are staring at my skin and my bandages – or, even worse, trying hard not to look – and it makes me feel very self-conscious. When I was at school I was always trying to get out of PE or swimming because I hated letting people see the patches of eczema that I normally covered up with long-sleeved clothes.

I find that it helps to explain exactly what is wrong. Even though eczema is so common, a lot of people don't seem to realize that it's not catching and has nothing to do with being dirty.

Like everyone else, people with eczema need the boost to their self-esteem that comes from being loved and cared about. It's important to remind yourself that *nobody is perfect* and that your friends and family love you just as you are. The NES suggests that you make a point of doing things that give you a feeling of achievement, take up challenges, and find interests and hobbies you enjoy and which absorb you. You are more than just your skin!

It really is worth experimenting to find the best way of dealing with your eczema. You'll need determination and patience. If one kind of emollient or steroid cream doesn't work for you, ask to try another. The relaxation techniques mentioned in the section on sleep problems are also helpful and we shall be going into 'complementary' therapies in greater detail in Chapter 8. Whatever relaxation technique works best for you, it's important to set time aside to practise it, however busy your life is.

Your family, friends and loved ones can help, partly by ensuring that you know they love you, whatever the state of your skin. As with any problem, it always helps to talk things over so that they can make allowances if you are sometimes irritable and snappy because you are being driven crazy by that persistent itch.

'I have physically held Chelsea's hands to stop her scratching,' admits mum Nina, 'but all she did was shout at me, "You don't know what it's like, I *have* to scratch."'

Many others, like Chelsea, often say that it doesn't help to be told not to scratch or be reminded to use their emollient as the chances are they have already thought of that – or that they wouldn't be scratching if they weren't driven to distraction by the itching. A comforting hug (if it's not too painful) can help, or a chat or the offer of some outing or game, or perhaps a piece of music or TV programme that might take their mind off their skin for a moment. It's sometimes hard to sympathize with someone with a chronic condition like eczema which comes and goes and doesn't seem to improve. However much you might want to help, what can you say?

A supportive partner is a big help, as one woman told the NES. 'At times I have felt like something from a horror film but my husband still tells me he loves me no matter how bad my skin looks or feels. I don't always believe him!'

Marion, who suffered from childhood eczema and still has flare-ups, agrees.

> I have found the whole experience of eczema had a big effect on my confidence and body image. Thankfully as I've got older I have become more at peace with my body. I am also very fortunate in having a wonderful partner who really doesn't care if, or when, I suffer from spots, eczema or the thinning skin I now have on my hands – he just loves and cares about the person within.

Because there is no one-size-fits-all cure for eczema, most people say it's worth giving almost anything a try, no matter how odd-sounding. When interviewing the people whose experiences are quoted above, I asked them what they had found most helpful and the answers were extremely varied.

'A friend recommended the Body Shop's Body Butters range,' said Nina, whose teenage daughter Chelsea has eczema on her hands, arms, elbows, face and sometimes her knees. 'Chelsea carries a tub of their Brazil Nut Butter around with her wherever she goes and it seems to suit her best out of the hundreds of things we have tried over the years.'

'Be your own health practitioner and find out what works and doesn't work for you,' advises Diane. 'You know more about your own skin than even your GP or dermatologist.'

'When I was a child, swimming in the sea always made my skin feel better,' says Marion, who is in her fifties. 'I don't use drugs because I prefer natural remedies and find that if I buy

Dead Sea salts and throw a handful into a bowl of water, it helps, even though it stings at the time. I am careful to dry my hands naturally, no rough towels, and I rarely have flare-ups now.'

Anne, also in her fifties, found an even more painful-sounding solution.

> The only treatment I found that worked was to bathe my sore arms with very hot water and then dab on neat Dettol. It hurt for a while but it did seem to stop the itching and also lessen the rash. I have also found a solid stick of witch hazel heals almost anything for me.

Ouch.

Eczema at work

As Diane says, having severe eczema can affect many less obvious aspects of your life, for instance the career you choose. If you have eczema as a child and you discover it is made worse by, for instance, contact with animal dander, or your skin reacts badly to everything but the gentlest skin cleansers or shampoos, then a career working with animals or one in hairdressing or the beauty business may not be the wisest choice for you. If cold weather leads to a flare-up, you will have to think twice about outdoor work like farming, forestry or horticulture. Alternatively, if heat is a problem for you, the warm, steamy atmosphere of a restaurant kitchen or a gym might not be the right environment for you to work in. Even work in an office, shop or factory can cause problems for those with eczema if they are exposed to a dusty atmosphere, direct sunlight or air-conditioning.

People with eczema do have to think 'outside the box' when career choices are being made. Nursing and any job involving patient care, for instance, means a lot of hand-washing, and latex gloves are often worn, so it could be an inappropriate choice. However, there may be another kind of healthcare job which might suit you, for instance occupational therapy. The National Eczema Society's leaflet 'Working with Eczema' lists career areas which could be problematic. As well as those already mentioned, they could include

- engineering or motor vehicle repair, because of contact with oils and coolants;
- building work, because contact with cement can cause irritation for some people, and allergy to chromate is common;
- work with adhesives containing cyanoacrylates and epoxy resins, both of which can cause allergic contact eczema.

The police and emergency services and the Armed Forces often raise a question mark when it comes to recruiting people with health problems like eczema. Firefighters and ambulance staff, for example, may find their work sometimes brings them into contact with chemicals. However, it does depend very much on how severe your eczema is and exactly what your job involves. The Metropolitan Police, for instance, say that every applicant is considered on a case-by-case basis and someone with eczema would only be ruled out if their condition affected their ability to do the job. Many of these careers require a medical check-up or filling in a health questionnaire and there are jobs in, for example, the Army or the ambulance service that someone with eczema would be able to do. The Health and Safety Executive say that no-one should be ruled out of any job if protective equipment – masks, gloves and/or other protective clothing – is available.

5

How your doctor can help

Because eczema is not a life-threatening condition, it doesn't get as much attention from the NHS and the media as other illnesses. Dermatology tends to be something of a 'Cinderella service', with the amount of help you can get depending on where you live and how much interest your own GP has in skin conditions.

When reporting to the House of Lords Science and Technology Committee on Allergy in October 2006, Allergy UK's Muriel Simmonds made the point that GPs receive very little training in the diagnosis and treatment of allergic conditions, including eczema. Many people contact Allergy UK in desperation, like the mum whose young son's skin was sore and bleeding. Her GP had brushed her aside and simply told her that she should continue to treat him with steroids, because allergy testing was a waste of time. Another GP refused to refer a seven-year-old with a sore skin and puffy eyes to a specialist, telling his mother that nothing could be done for him.

'We need more training for GPs,' says Ms Simmonds. 'Without properly diagnosed NHS patients, there can be no basic research, clinical trials or, importantly, research on NHS service delivery.'

Hospital dermatology departments provide a holistic approach to the management of eczema, often using clinics which are led by specialist nurses. Moira Craig, a dermatology nurse who is responsible for the skin clinic at Hillingdon Hospital in west London, agrees that GPs don't receive a great deal of training in dermatology.

'Eczema and psoriasis are the most common conditions I see,' she comments. 'Most major hospitals have dermatology departments, but there are few beds for dermatology patients. We tend to see patients who have had eczema for a long time.'

The problem is that the average GP consultation lasts about ten minutes. That isn't always long enough for you to discuss the problem, the GP to make a diagnosis, and for a treatment regime to be recommended that you can understand. Whether you are seeing your GP or you have been referred to a specialist clinic, it's always a good idea to jot down a list of questions you want to ask and to make notes about your treatment. This is especially important in the case of eczema, because *how* you use the creams and lotions your doctor prescribes is extremely important. You may be prescribed a soap substitute, a couple of different emollients, a special shampoo and bandages, and it can be confusing if you are not sure in what order to use them or how much of each product you need to use.

'Patients want to feel that they are in control,' says Moira Craig.

I always go through their existing skincare regime with them. To advise them properly, I will need to know what makes their eczema worse and whether they have a family history of allergic conditions, in order to establish what sort of eczema they have – whether, for instance, it is true atopic eczema or contact dermatitis.

Then I ask them what they use on their skin as a moisturizer and whether their doctor has prescribed anything. A surprising number of GPs don't even tell their patients not to use soap. I ask them how often they wash, bath or shower and what they use, whether they like very hot water, and how they use any creams. Some patients rub cream into their skin quite roughly and even use rough towels which may make the itching and soreness worse.

Patients don't always take in what they have been told, whether by me or by their doctor or pharmacist. When they do find out exactly how the creams they have been prescribed should be used, I often hear them say, 'Why didn't anyone tell me this before?'

Whatever kind of treatment you are prescribed, it's important to remember that it is unlikely to 'cure' your eczema. What treatment prescribed by your doctor or dermatologist does do is enable you to *manage* the condition. It's important to accept that and not feel disappointed that your doctor can't provide a miracle cure.

Emollient therapy

Most cases of eczema are treated initially by what is called 'emollient therapy' and many people find that when it's used properly this is a very effective way of controlling their eczema. Indeed, many people find they don't need anything else.

Emollients are creams, ointments, gels, lotions, bath oils and soap substitutes, made from a mixture of fats, oils and water, which are used in place of ordinary soaps, detergents and bath products. Because dry, itchy, sensitive skin lacks normal moisture, this has to be replaced by the moisture in emollient products, which has a soothing and protective effect. We saw in Chapter 1 that the stratum corneum, the outermost layer of the skin, exists to prevent water loss from the skin as well as preventing irritants, allergens and infections penetrating the inner layers. When eczema develops and the skin becomes dry and cracked, emollients are prescribed to provide an oily, moist layer on the surface of the stratum corneum. This traps water underneath it, moisturizing the skin, and also prevents the irritants, allergens and infections penetrating the deeper layers of the skin.

There are several different ranges of emollients on the market so if the one you are first prescribed doesn't suit you, ask if you can try something else. Dermatology clinics like Moira Craig's can offer samples of different brands to people, so that they can find out which suits them best by trial and error. Information on individual emollient ranges is obtainable from the manufacturers and also from the NES. Many emollients have ranges which are specially formulated for use on children. Your GP or pharmacist may also be able to answer any questions you may have.

Generally, the advice is to use plenty of emollient, smoothing it into the skin rather than rubbing, and to replace all your usual toiletries and moisturizing creams with emollients to give your skin the best possible chance. Use plenty of emollient in your bath, making sure that the water is not too hot. Follow the instructions on the pack which will tell you just how much to use. Stay in the bath for 10–20 minutes to give the emollient time to soak into your skin. Pat your body dry gently and take care not to rub all the emollient off, as it leaves a film which has a protective effect. You can use gel on damp skin, after a bath or shower, and the cream or ointment you have been prescribed as often as you feel you need it, whenever your skin is feeling especially dry or irritated. As a guideline, it is suggested that you apply emollient every four hours or at least three or four times per day.

For the more severe forms of eczema, a technique called 'wet-wrapping' is a way of ensuring that the skin benefits from as much emollient as possible. It's especially suitable for those whose eczema is most troublesome on their arms and legs, but (especially in children) it is possible to 'wet-wrap' the whole body. The basic method involves applying a thick layer of emollient (and sometimes a layer of mild or moderately potent steroid; see the following section). This is then topped with a layer of wet bandages, followed by another layer of dry bandages, which can be worn overnight and also through the daytime if necessary. Many people find this soothing, but you will probably need help from a specialist to show you how best to do it.

Dermatology nurse Moira Craig explains that it's a false economy to skimp on your use of emollients.

> Pharmacists and GPs sometimes differ in the advice they give. Some advise patients to apply emollients sparingly though dermatologists recommend slapping it on. Most emollients are available without prescription but when you can be using as much as one 500 gm tub per week they can seem expensive. For those with long-term eczema problems I would suggest you get a pre-paid annual prescription as that can work out more economical.

In addition to prescribing emollients, your GP will encourage you to identify and avoid any of the 'triggers' which cause your eczema to flare up. It isn't always easy to identify your own triggers but you could keep an 'eczema diary' and note what was happening when your flare-ups occurred. Was the weather especially cold, or hot? Had you started using a different kind of detergent or worn more woolly jumpers or artificial fabrics next to your skin? Had the family acquired a new pet, or have you visited, or been visited by, a pet-owner? Had you been under particular stress? Had you changed your diet? Experience should teach you what your triggers are so that you can adapt your lifestyle to avoid them as far as possible.

The truth about steroids

If a combination of avoiding your personal eczema triggers and using plenty of suitable emollient doesn't seem enough to get your troublesome skin under control, the next step is often the prescription of topical steroids.

There is a lot of misunderstanding about these drugs and their use. Part of the problem is that the topical steroids prescribed for skin conditions are often confused with the anabolic steroids used (and sometimes misused) by body-builders, although they are not the same drugs. Corticosteroids, to give them their full name, are similar to the natural hormones produced by the body's adrenal glands, which are situated just above the kidneys.

These hormones regulate the balance of mineral salts and the water content of the body. In larger amounts, they can reduce inflammation and suppress allergic reactions.

Topical steroids are drugs specially formulated for use on the skin. They come in a range of strengths or 'potencies' and in the form of creams, lotions and ointments. Most are available on prescription only, except for the very mildest 1 per cent hydrocortisone cream, which you can buy over the counter from your pharmacist. It's normally used to treat the irritation arising from insect bites or mild contact dermatitis. Steroids work by preventing the release of the chemicals that trigger inflammation in the skin.

Moderate, potent or very potent steroids can only be prescribed by your doctor and are used to bring severe skin flare-ups under control quickly and effectively. Normally they are used for only a short time, especially the more potent steroids. Because eczema is a condition which can flare up at intervals, some people find that they need a short course of a more potent steroid preparation from time to time, and that when their skin condition is controlled they can manage it by using a milder steroid or possibly emollients alone.

Your GP will decide which steroid to prescribe, taking into account factors like your age and the condition of your skin. You will usually be prescribed a mild steroid first, and only if that doesn't prove effective will your doctor change the prescription to a more potent preparation. The more potent versions are not suitable for facial use. Steroids should always be used according to directions, either from your doctor or from the patient information leaflet in the packet.

People are often concerned about being prescribed steroids, especially for use on children. However, these drugs have been used in the treatment of skin conditions like eczema for more than thirty years and have a generally good safety record. Like all drugs, though, they can have side-effects and are not suitable for everyone. The most common side-effect is thinning of the skin, but this normally only happens after prolonged use of the more potent steroids. Facial skin is most susceptible to this effect which is why only the weaker steroids are prescribed for use on the face. However, for short-term use to control an eczema flare-up, steroids are perfectly safe for most people, including children.

'Steroids have had a bad press and I have spoken to patients who are worried about skin damage and weight gain when taking them,' comments dermatology nurse Moira Craig.

> Modern steroids are improving all the time, and they are a useful treatment for damaged skin in the short term. I always remind my patients that there is a risk of skin damage from conditions like eczema if you *don't* use steroids. People with damaged skin are also much more vulnerable to bacterial infections like staphylococcus aureus and MRSA.

The NES advises care, when using steroids, to make sure you are using the correct amount, and reminds people that they should also be using emollients, allowing at least 30 minutes between applying steroid cream and applying an emollient. They provide the following guidelines for steroid use:

- Don't use topical steroids on facial skin unless your doctor has told you to.
- Do tell your doctor if you are pregnant or planning to become pregnant.
- Don't use steroids for longer than you are told to.
- Do go back to your GP if there is no improvement in your skin in two weeks.
- Do contact your doctor for advice if your skin gets worse while using a steroid (you may be allergic to this drug, or have an infection).
- Don't use steroids which have been prescribed for someone else, as they may be an inappropriate strength and unsuitable for your skin.

The British Skin Foundation also has what it calls 'Golden Rules' for steroid use which you might find helpful. They include:

- Use the weakest possible cream that maintains good control of your eczema.
- Use ointment rather than creams if possible, as ointment tends to stay on the skin longer, and this helps the active ingredient to work.
- Use preparations for short periods (10–14 days is suggested) followed by 'emollient holidays'.
- Use steroid cream or ointment along with your usual emollient. They suggest you allow one hour between applying steroid ointment and emollient as the emollient can otherwise dilute the effect of the steroid. (This is a longer interval than the NES recommend. If a half-hour gap doesn't seem to improve the condition of your skin, try leaving a longer interval.)
- Used sensibly, steroids do not cause side-effects. Untreated eczema can have serious consequences for the skin.
- Get more of your prescribed preparation from your GP when the tube you are using is one-quarter full. Take the old tubes along to the doctor so that she can monitor how much you are using.

Other drug treatments

Emollients and steroids are the longest-established and best-researched treatments for eczema, but there are other drugs which can be prescribed. Some of these are especially useful for those whose eczema does not respond to the more usual treatments.

Anti-histamines, especially those which have a sedative effect, are sometimes prescribed to help reduce the 'itch–scratch' cycle and allow people with eczema to get some sleep. While people are sleeping they can't scratch and this gives their skin a chance to 'cool down' and even heal. Researchers have also been studying one of the drugs normally prescribed to treat hay fever and allergic conjunctivitis, Nalcrom, otherwise known as sodium cromoglycate. This is a 'mast cell stabilizer' but so far there hasn't been any research which suggests it is an effective treatment for eczema.

Another drug sometimes prescribed to relieve the itching is doxepin hydrochloride or *Xepin cream*. It is not known how this works, and it is only recommended for use on small areas of skin. If it's used in large amounts it can cause side-effects like drowsiness. Xepin cream is not normally used to treat children under 12.

If the skin becomes infected by bacteria or fungi, shown by crusting, weeping or a sudden worsening of the soreness, your doctor will probably prescribe a course of *antibiotics* or *antifungals*. Both can come in the form of creams, tablets or capsules and are only recommended for short-term use, until the infection clears up.

Severe eczema which is not sufficiently controlled by emollients and steroids is sometimes treated with another class of drugs, the *immunosuppressants*, notably cyclosporin. These are drugs, usually taken as tablets or capsules, which are used to suppress the body's natural defences against infection. For example, they are often prescribed to patients after organ transplants, when there's a danger of the body rejecting the new organ. However, they have also been found useful in treating severe skin conditions when more usual treatments like steroids have not helped.

Like all drugs, cyclosporin can cause side-effects, including nausea, increased body hair and occasionally kidney or liver damage, so it's important that you are carefully monitored if you're taking this drug. People who are taking immunosuppressants are also, naturally, more at risk of developing infections so should take special care to stay healthy. Because of possible side-effects, cyclosporin is normally only prescribed for short-term use.

More recently, two new topical immunomodulator drugs, tacrolimus (Protopic) and pimecrolimus (Elidel), have been introduced. If you find that topical steroids don't suit you, one of these drugs may be prescribed as an alternative as they don't seem to cause the same side-effects. They are especially useful in the treatment of facial eczema, when the use of potent steroid creams is not appropriate.

Elidel is a cream which can be useful in treating mild to moderate eczema, and is suitable for those over two years old. Protopic is an ointment which comes in two strengths, is used for treating moderate to severe eczema and, again, is suitable for those over two years old. These are the first new topical treatments for eczema to be introduced since topical steroids and they seem to work well, although as with any relatively new drug their long-term effects are not known. So far, the only reported side-effects seem to be a burning feeling and some reddening of the skin when the cream or ointment is first applied. This does not last long. The European Medicines Agency has warned that there may be a greater risk of skin cancer or lymphoma (another kind of cancer) in those who use these drugs, though as far as is known the benefits outweigh the risks.

Ultra-violet light treatment

You may have seen advertisements for clinics which treat eczema and other skin conditions with ultra-violet light (UVA). It is sometimes used on its own, or sometimes with the addition of a drug called psoralen (PUVA). Psoralen comes in the form of tablets, or as a solution which you add to bath water.

The British Association of Dermatologists say that there is a relatively small amount of reliable research into the efficacy of this kind of treatment. Doctors began to try it when they realized that many people found their eczema was less trouble-some in the summer, when they were exposed to sunlight. It's also known that ultra-violet light can help to treat psoriasis, another uncomfortable skin condition.

A few small research studies did find that short courses of UVA treatment benefited some people with eczema. There have not been reliable studies of PUVA treatment.

We already know that ultra-violet light can damage the skin, especially if people are exposed to it on a long-term basis – hence all the warnings about the risks of sunbeds and excessive sunbathing, which is linked to a much higher risk of developing skin cancer. Anyone who is already at higher risk of skin cancer – fair-skinned and freckled people with a lot of skin blemishes and moles, for example, or those with skin cancer in the family – might be better avoiding this kind of treatment. If you are considering it, ask your GP or dermatologist's advice.

The people with eczema I spoke to for this book reported very variable results from the existing range of GP-prescribed treatments. Marion, for example, was put on steroids in her mid-teens to deal with the eczema she had had since childhood and found they were extremely effective, although she says they did cause some skin thinning. Anne found steroids did not help at all, and Diane, whose eczema is extremely severe, says that she no longer uses them because she believes they cause too much damage to already thin skin.

Sian used a combination of emollients, very mild steroids, diet and lifestyle changes to treat her seven-year-old son Simon, with considerable success.

> We did attend a specialist allergy clinic, fortunately. I have heard lots of stories of people just handed a prescription and not told exactly how to use emollients or steroids properly. What worked for Simon was ensuring his skin was scrupulously clean, applying the 1 per cent hydrocortisone cream, waiting 15 minutes, then adding the emollient. Patients really need to be shown how to use it all properly: that could make the differ-ence between the treatment working and not working.

6

Lifestyle changes

In addition to emollient therapy and the use of steroids or other drugs to treat eczema, most people seem at least to try and experiment with what are known as 'lifestyle changes' to see if their skin condition improves. That can mean anything from using only specially formulated or organic toiletries to re-furnishing the house with wooden or laminate floors and leather furniture in place of dusty carpets and upholstery.

The trouble is, there isn't a lot of convincing scientific evidence that any of this works – although, annoyingly, *some* lifestyle changes seem to work for *some* people. If you know what triggers an eczema flare-up in your particular case, obviously it makes sense to avoid it. When I was speaking to people with eczema for this book, the phrase 'trial and error' came up over and over again. Most try to wear pure cotton clothing, with artificial fabrics a no-no. They also said they avoided soap and biological washing powders. Many have become sceptical of the claims made for various products.

'We must have spent hundreds of pounds over the years and none of the creams and potions we tried really made much difference,' says Nina, mum of 14-year-old Chelsea.

I also spoke to two leading dermatologists. One of them, Professor Julia Newton Bishop, who runs the paediatric eczema clinic at St James's University Hospital, Leeds, told me that she believes eczema to be

a genetic condition with environmental issues. That being so, it makes sense to keep sensitive skin away from known irritants like wool, seams and clothes labels. Some people are badly affected by the house-dust mite. A few do seem to benefit from total allergen avoidance, though on the whole the evidence for this is fairly weak.

Sensible and cheap options would include putting a cotton throw over the sofa, or even on the floor when there are small children around. Crawling babies can get eczema on their knees. Washing cotton fabrics at 60 degrees seems to help, but none of these measures will necessarily benefit everyone.

Fellow skin expert Sue Lewis-Jones, Consultant Dermatologist at Ninewells Hospital, Dundee, says that most lifestyle changes seem to be based on house-dust mite avoidance.

> This is very important in cases of asthma, and can help some people with eczema too. The trouble is that in an ordinary home it is hard to reduce allergen levels enough to make a difference. Eczema seems to have multi-factorial causes so if you change three things in your home – say the type of clothes you wear, the bedding or the flooring – there could easily be another three that are still left to cause you problems.

Both dermatologists recommend the simple, easy, inexpensive changes you can make. As well as those mentioned above, they can include: minimizing the number of soft furnishings, cushions and so on you have in the house; popping your child's soft toys in the freezer overnight to kill the house-dust mites; discarding dusty old carpets and feather pillows; using non-biological washing powders; and letting someone else mow the lawn!

About house-dust mites

These little creatures, or rather their droppings, are the enemy of anyone who suffers from any kind of allergic condition. However clean your home, there will be house-dust mites in it. House-dust mites have a life cycle of up to three months. In that time, a female can lay as many as 300 eggs! Modern houses, with their central heating, fitted carpets and thick insulation, are a perfect breeding ground for them to survive and thrive.

Invisible to the naked eye, they live in our soft furnishings, including bedding and upholstery. A mattress can contain as many as 10,000 dust mites and 2 million dust-mite droppings. Allergy UK say that we all lose something like 87 litres of sweat and 500 g of dead skin over the course of a year. Our beds are the ideal environment for dust mites, which can cause allergic reactions – not just eczema – in up to 85 per cent of people affected.

Removing dust mites from your home completely is virtually impossible but you can keep the numbers down. Once you have established your eczema is triggered by being in a dusty atmosphere, here are some suggestions you might consider:

- Turn down the central heating a little and make sure that your home is well ventilated.
- Change your carpets and rugs for other types of flooring – wood, laminate, cork, tiles or fashionable rubber. There is an organization called the Healthy Flooring Network (for contact details see Useful addresses) which can give you more information.
- Vacuum your floors regularly with a high-filtration vacuum cleaner. Cleaners with an HEPA filter are now widely available. Dyson, for example, make a range of cleaners which have the Allergy UK Seal of Approval.
- Replace heavy curtains, which can become very dusty, with wooden or vinyl wipe-clean blinds.
- When the time comes to replace your old sofa or suite, think about leather or rattan rather than upholstery.
- Dust with a damp cloth rather than an old-fashioned duster, which is inclined to spread the dust from place to place.
- Reduce the humidity levels in your home as far as is practical. If you are doing the washing, keep the kitchen or utility-room door closed to avoid spreading damp air to the rest of the house. Dry clothes out of doors rather than on radiators. Keep

relative humidity below 50 per cent – you can buy a hygrometer at hardware stores to measure it.

- Take a look at some of the anti-allergy bedding on the market. High-street stores like John Lewis have suitable ranges and there are many specialist companies like The Healthy House Ltd and AllergyBestBuys (see Useful addresses) selling it by mail order or via the Internet. The NES can give you more details of companies selling this type of product.
- Replace pillows every 18 months and duvets every three to five years.
- Experiment with some of the sprays, such as Total Hygiene DM-1 Spray (see Useful addresses), which can be used on soft furnishings as well as carpets and curtains.

Indoor air pollution

The contribution which air pollution – both indoor and outdoor – has made to the rise of allergic conditions like eczema in the last twenty or thirty years is still being debated. As yet, the jury is still out. There doesn't seem to be any firm evidence that either air pollution, for instance from car exhaust fumes, or the number of chemicals present in our homes is to blame. Many companies advertise 'air cleaners' 'air purifiers' and 'air ionizers' which claim to remove chemicals from the home and make the air we breathe healthier, although dermatologists I spoke to were sceptical about the value of these products. They are also quite expensive (£350–£450) and can be noisy.

All the same, it is unnerving to realize just what might be in the cocktail of chemicals we breathe in every day and to know that there could be ten times as much pollution inside our homes as there is in the street outside! Pesticides, flame retardants, solvents, the cleaners and sprays and detergents you use in the kitchen, the bathroom and the garden are all thought to be harmless in the small amounts normally used. But do they contribute to your eczema, and if they do, are there alternatives?

The first thing to remember is that even if a product is labelled 'natural' and/or 'organic' that doesn't necessarily mean that it will not irritate your skin. There are plenty of natural skin irritants, such as poison ivy. However, if you want to avoid chemical-based products, others are available. The best-known range is Ecover, which is widely available from supermarkets, and which includes washing powders and liquids, stain removers, and cleaners for toilets, floors, bathrooms and ovens. Other names to look out for include Bio-D, which you can find in health food shops. All their products are allergy tested as well as being environmentally friendly. Almost all the people with eczema I spoke to when I was researching this book told me that avoiding biological washing powders seemed to help their skin condition.

If you are a DIY-er, or married to one, you might well find that your eczema is made much worse when you're decorating or carrying out home improvements. Just looking at a list of ingredients on a tin of paint or solvent can be worrying. Some manufacturers are now labelling paints and other products as 'lower in VOCs' (volatile organic compounds) and these are worth looking out for. There are also special ranges of 'natural' paints and other products made from traditional materials available from companies like the Green Building Store in West Yorkshire. The Healthy House catalogue also carries a good range of Ecos organic paints (see Useful addresses for contact details).

Clothing

Natural fibres like silk and cotton seem to suit most sensitive skins – although wool, which is of course a natural fibre, can be extremely irritating if worn next to the skin. According to the NES, there are many companies which make suitable clothing for people with eczema, especially children. Many are small businesses set up by families whose own children suffered badly from the condition and who were unable to find anything suitable, comfortable and also stylish for them to wear.

The Healthy House carries a small range of children's organic cotton clothing, including T-shirts, pyjamas, leggings and mitten suits which prevent children from scratching. They are specially made with flat seams to be as non-irritating as possible. The company also sells cotton gloves in both children's and adults' sizes.

Pure Cotton Comfort is one of the companies started by a young mother whose daughter suffered from eczema. It now offers a range of appropriate clothing for both children and adults, including pyjamas suitable for those with severe eczema to help to break the itch–scratch cycle. Adult clothing includes 100 per cent untreated cotton underwear for both men and women, nightwear, socks and tights. (For contact details see Useful addresses.)

Cosmetics and toiletries

The trend towards natural and organic products seems to be most pronounced in the world of cosmetics, with even major manufacturers falling over themselves to give their products a 'natural' label. However, as with other products, 'natural' doesn't necessarily mean that those with eczema will find them suitable. I have spoken to people who had bad reactions to 'natural' lavender hand cream and also to Tea Tree Oil.

Having said that, it is most noticeable that many of the highly successful, smaller cosmetic companies like Green People (for contact details see Useful addresses) were started by women who either could not use conventional cosmetics and toiletries themselves or whose children were unable to. Charlotte Vohtz, founder of Green People, is a case in point. As Charlotte says:

It all began with a two-year-old girl who couldn't stop scratching herself. My daughter Sandra suffered from severe eczema and allergies. She came out in a rash every time she touched any kind of shampoo, shower gel, soap or skin product.

Charlotte treated her daughter with a herbal elixir and organic essential fatty acids which helped her skin problems, and replaced all their carpets with wooden, stone and tiled floors. As a former nurse and medical researcher, she was horrified to discover how many man-made chemicals are used in personal care products – even in some of those labelled 'natural' – and set about researching and developing formulations which were safe, gentle and effective in use. This is how Green People began in 1997. They now have a range of more than a hundred skin and personal care products for men, women and children, plus a small range of household products.

Grandma Vine's is another range of products which some people find helpful, particularly their Antiseptic Gel. Free from petrochemicals and animal products, colourings and harsh preservatives, this product soothes dry, itchy skin as well as helping to heal cuts and grazes. As one satisfied customer says,

I have had eczema for 15 years and have used a variety of creams and gels supplied by my doctor. Grandma Vine's Antiseptic Gel works more effectively than any prescription to date. When I applied the gel the results were immediate. When my eczema flares up it usually takes three or four days to bring it under control. With the gel, I need only apply once at bedtime and it has cleared up by morning.

Margaret Weeds, whose company Essential Care is based in Suffolk (for contact details see Useful addresses), is another mother who began formulating her own range of skincare products because of eczema, allergies and sensitive skin in her family. Other names to look out for include Weleda, whose range includes Dermatodoron Ointment, specially formulated as a treatment to manage chronic eczema. The Jurlique range of skincare products, founded by a German naturopath and formulated from plants grown on his Australian organic and biodynamic farm, is also suitable for highly sensitive skins.

Another Australian product, called Hope's Relief Cream (for contact details see Useful addresses), got glowing reviews in the *Guardian*'s 'Family' section in early 2007.

Oat-based products suit some people; names to look out for include A-Derma and Aveeno. A cheap way to find out whether this helps your skin is to put some ordinary porridge oats into a piece of muslin and soak them in your bath, making sure you squeeze the 'oat milk' out. It can be very soothing.

You should be aware, however, that there is no absolute guarantee that any of these products will *not* cause a problem for your sensitive skin. Jurlique suggest that when trying any new skincare product, you start by applying a small amount to an area of about 2 sq cm on your inner forearm. If you don't experience any adverse reaction, you can try using it on another part of your body and then, cautiously, on your face. They also recommend that you try new products one at a time, so that your skin doesn't have too many unfamiliar products to cope with at once and that if you do suffer from a flare-up, you can identify the culprit easily.

Having said that, some people with eczema say that they can use high-street brands of cosmetics and skincare products with no problem. It really does seem to be a case of trying out the products first.

Pets

It's quite common for people to find that their eczema is triggered by any contact with pets, especially cats and dogs. Some are so sensitive that they begin to itch if they are in close contact with a pet-owner or go into a house where there is a pet, even when the animal isn't there. Contrary to popular belief, it's not the pet fur that causes the problem, it's 'dander', which is the mixture of hair and saliva present on an animal's coat after it has groomed itself.

The solution would appear to be simple: if animals trigger your eczema, don't keep furry or feathered pets. It can be hard to avoid other people's, though. A product called Petal Cleanse (which comes in two formulas, one for dogs and one for cats) is said to be effective in removing dander and minimizing allergic responses (for contact details see Bio-Life Europe Ltd in Useful addresses). Outright Allergy Relief products (see Useful addresses) are also available from pet shops. If you have problems with animals and your children are nagging you for a pet, see if you can persuade them to develop an interest in keeping tropical fish, stick insects or even giant African land snails!

Does stress make your eczema worse?

Having an unpredictable chronic condition like eczema can be stressful in itself. A survey of callers to the National Eczema Society revealed that 88 per cent of them said that stress could trigger their eczema or make it worse. Carers and family members of those with eczema can also find the condition stressful. You can't be sure when you are going to have a flare-up and you always hope that special occasions like family weddings or school exams are not going to be affected by an uncomfortable, itchy skin.

Fourteen-year-old Chelsea says she has noticed that her eczema is worse if she is stressed or upset about anything.

> School exams, rows with Mum and Dad, and when I changed schools I had a really bad flare-up which made me feel very self-conscious. I used to worry a lot more about it when I first went to secondary school but I have a really good crowd of friends who accept me just the way I am, and I am definitely more relaxed about my eczema than I used to be. I don't know if it's coincidence but I don't get as many flare-ups either.

If you suspect your eczema flare-ups could be stress-related, the old suggestion to keep an eczema diary is a good one. The NES also recommends that, instead of letting your eczema raise your stress levels – which then aggravate your eczema, which then raises your stress levels still more – you should

- identify the sources of stress you can avoid;
- find better ways of dealing with the unavoidable stress in your life;
- and, above all, make sure your eczema is being treated appropriately.

Many people, not just those with eczema, feel stressed when they don't seem to be in control of their lives. You will need to remember that you are in charge of your eczema, rather than letting it control you! Get all the help you can from your GP or dermatology nurse and don't be afraid to experiment with the different products and lifestyle changes discussed in this chapter. They don't all work for everyone but some of them may work for you. Then at least you will feel you are doing all you can to help yourself.

Everyone can benefit from learning a relaxation technique. This might mean going to formal classes in yoga, meditation, visualization, autogenic training or t'ai chi, or just finding your own personal 'switch-off' technique. We'll be looking at complementary therapies like yoga in more detail in Chapter 8. Relaxation CDs and DVDs are widely available, some no more than gentle soothing music, others offering 'guided visualizations' which you may find helpful. Your personal favourite piece of classical music could work just as well. A warm bath with a glass of wine, a candle-lit supper, an absorbing novel ... anything that enables you to take a break from your hectic life can help to relax you. Massage and aromatherapy are extremely soothing, though you need to be careful that you don't use products which irritate your skin and if it is very sore massage may be inappropriate anyway. If things are getting you down and you don't feel you can confide in friends or family, you might benefit from counselling.

You will be much better able to cope with stress if your general health is good, so make sure you are eating sensibly and getting plenty of healthy exercise. Did you know that your blood pressure drops by a few points as soon as you start to walk under trees? Any kind of exercise helps to release endorphins, the body's feel-good hormones, so find something you enjoy doing and promise yourself you'll spare half an hour every day to get your body moving.

Are you getting enough sleep? It is very much easier to cope with the stresses and strains of daily life if you are getting a good night's sleep – but are you? Most people suffer from insomnia at some time, and up to a third of us claim to be chronic poor sleepers. Much insomnia is caused by stress and anxiety – and ironically, the less well you sleep the more anxious and stressed you are likely to be! Lack of sleep has a general stress effect on the body with rising levels of the stress hormone cortisol in the bloodstream.

There's no 'right amount' of sleep for everyone. Sleep experts say that if you wake up refreshed and ready for the day ahead, you are getting enough sleep whether you've been in bed for four hours or nine. Sleeping pills can only ever be a short-term answer to insomnia. Many of the relaxation therapies mentioned in Chapter 8 should help if you have trouble sleeping.

Simple ways to reduce the stress in your life

There are as many ways of winding down from everyday stress as there are people! For some, even the daily commute can be a stress-buster rather than a stress-inducer, as 51-year-old Laura explains.

I have a half-hour drive to the office every day. Instead of using the dual carriageway I make a point of travelling along country roads. I have a

CD player in my car and I put on some favourite music and just sing along. My mobile is switched off and I think of that half-hour as 'me' time, when neither my husband, my two teenagers nor my colleagues at work can reach me. Modern communications mean we are now expected to be in touch at all times but I think that's a recipe for stress. If they can't manage without me for half an hour, morning and evening, it's just too bad!

Laura's attitude is a healthy one. So many people simply try to do too much – both at work and at home – instead of learning a few basic time-management skills that would enable them to cope better with the demands of the day. If you feel stressed because life is getting on top of you and there never seem to be quite enough hours in the day, try sitting down and making a list of all the things you have to do

- today;
- this week;
- in the next six months.

Today's list could include doing the laundry, going to work, shopping for tonight's dinner in your lunch hour, meeting a friend after work, taking your daughter to Brownies, cooking dinner, writing a report for work, walking the dog, writing and posting a birthday card for your mum, washing your hair.

This week's list could include the rest of the housework, a major shop, ironing, booking a dental appointment, taking the car for its MOT, introducing a new member of staff at work to her schedule, going out to dinner with friends.

The 'six-months' list could include applying for promotion, choosing and booking your holiday, getting something done about the leaking roof, tidying the garden, planning the new kitchen you've been dreaming of, arranging a surprise party for your partner's birthday ... and so on and so on.

Now, look at those lists again. Are you surprised you're feeling stressed? Borrow the kids' coloured crayons and put red stars by all the tasks you absolutely have to do, and blue crosses by the ones someone else could do perfectly well. That will leave you with some which – whisper it –*don't have to be done at all*. Stop trying to be a superwoman or superman. There's no such thing, and you will run yourself ragged even attempting it. All household tasks can be shared, and no one wants to live on a film-set anyway. Similarly, many work tasks can be better organized, or delegated to someone else.

Stress-busters

There are plenty of books on household management and quick cooking for busy women. Once you have off-loaded some of the unnecessary demands on your time, how are you going to use it to de-stress properly? Quick, easy, everyday stress-busters can include:

- Laughter: it has been proved that laughter can banish stress, so watch a comedy DVD.
- Pets in your life: we can all learn a lot about relaxation by watching a sleeping cat. Dentists sometimes have tanks of tropical fish in their waiting-rooms to calm nervous people's fears.
- Plants and flowers: scientific studies have shown that hospital patients recover more quickly when they can see trees from their ward window, and blood pressure drops when people walk in woodlands.
- An absorbing hobby: men seem to be better at what is sometimes known as 'the potting-shed syndrome' when they switch off from everyday worries by retiring to the potting shed. Golf and gardening play the same de-stressing role. Isn't there something you could become just as absorbed in – a craft like pottery, an amateur dramatic group or choir, a col-

lection that gets you rooting about for bargains in junk shops and car-boot sales?

- A sense of perspective: many of the everyday things that wind us up and raise our blood pressure are not really *that* important. When you feel your stress levels rising, ask yourself how much it really matters that you're stuck at a red traffic-light or you've had to wait ages in a bank or supermarket queue. That's the time to take a few deep, relaxing breaths, let those tense shoulders drop, and take yourself to ...
- A 'happy place': there must be somewhere – a favourite holiday beach, your own comfortable bed, an armchair by the fire – where you feel completely relaxed. When things get too much for you, close your eyes and imagine you're there. Feel the sand between your toes or the warmth of the blankets, listen to the waves or the crackling of the flames. Imagine your toddler's toothy grin, your partner's arms round you, your cat purring on your lap, and feel the tension drain away.

True relaxation isn't something you can learn overnight. Just as with eczema treatments, there are no instant quick-fixes. Give yourself time, a bit of private space that's free from interruptions (close the door, switch off the phone) and let those worries float away ...

7

Eczema and diet

If you have read this far in the book, you'll be aware that there are no instant answers or one-size-fits-all treatments or cures for eczema. Nowhere is that more evident than in the area of eczema and diet. The official line seems to be that relatively few cases of eczema can be helped by a change of diet – especially in adults – although most of the eczema cases I spoke to for this book said there were things they just couldn't eat, and one or two said that what is known as 'dietary manipulation' had made a real difference.

Roz, 30, said,

> I've had both eczema and asthma for over twenty-five years, since I was five. I have only just discovered that I am allergic to cow's milk, and it was the milk, butter, cream, cheese and other dairy products that I had been eating which caused my bad skin, wheezing and runny nose. I would recommend anyone with any kind of allergic problem to try completely giving up cow's milk for a few weeks to see if it helps. It has completely changed my life.

Whether or not you discover a food allergy or intolerance, eating well is always helpful for any chronic health condition. That means following general guidelines like eating at least five portions of fruit and vegetables per day, cutting down on saturated fats and processed foods, and drinking plenty of water. Registered dietician Emma Mills offers nutritional advice to those with eczema and points out that although the right diet is unlikely to cure eczema in itself, it can help you manage the condition, alongside other factors like emollients.

> Your nutritional state has an impact on all areas of your health. Certain dietary factors can significantly influence inflammatory

conditions, including eczema. Medical interventions and emollient creams will not achieve maximum efficacy in someone who is poorly nourished. My opinion is that a nutrient-rich diet is vital for all individuals suffering from eczema.

Emma agrees that in babies and children, eczema can be associated with food allergy or food intolerance, and that many children grow out of it as their immune system matures. She underlines the importance of a healthy, balanced diet for growing children and believes that 'exclusion diets' should only be tried under the supervision of a paediatric dietician.

> People often don't realize that the right nutrients have a huge impact on the way the brain and body work. Being on a very restrictive diet may affect a child's growth or development unless it is very carefully worked out. Natural, home-cooked meals with plenty of vegetables, fish and wholegrains give children the best basis for good health. If children come to the table hungry because they haven't been given between-meal snacks, they will eat what's put in front of them. You need to lead by example and eat with your children. It may sound old-fashioned, but it works.

A properly worked-out diet can have a huge impact on childhood eczema, as Sian discovered. Her young son Simon suffered really badly from eczema as a baby. He was referred to a specialist allergy clinic when he was just under six months old.

> I was feeding him myself and topping-up with milk formula. However, the tests they did at the clinic showed that he was allergic to cow's milk so I started giving him a special hypo-allergenic formula called Nutramigen. Some paediatric allergy specialists won't do tests on babies because they aren't always accurate but they were very accurate in Simon's case. He tested positive for egg, fish and corn as well as milk. When I began weaning him I found all these things upset his tummy, but only milk seemed to trigger his eczema.
>
> As soon as we changed his diet, his skin improved. As he grew, he was able to tolerate more foods. I was still using emollients and hydrocortisone cream as well, and by the time he went to nursery at three, his skin was clear apart from the occasional flare-up.

Then I heard about some Scandinavian research into probiotics as a treatment for eczema and bought a probiotic powder which I mixed with his Nutramigen. I didn't expect to see much of a change but within two weeks his skin was smooth, like a young child's should be. All the rough patches and redness behind his knees had gone.

Simon is seven now and still taking probiotics. He hardly ever gets a flare-up. His younger brother, aged two and a half, had mild eczema too but when I started him on the probiotics the eczema disappeared. Our local skin specialist tells parents to try good probiotics, although I know not all eczema is diet-related, even in children. It worked for us!

There does seem to be more information about diet manipulation in childhood than in adult eczema, and this is where most research is taking place. Unfortunately, what research there is tends to be inconclusive and sometimes contradictory.

'The literature on the subject is confusing,' agrees leading dermatologist Julia Newton Bishop.

Research in the USA has found that dietary changes can make a difference to many very young children – under a year old – and research at Great Ormond Street has also found that some babies do benefit. From my own observations, cow's milk and egg avoidance can help but as yet there is no real scientific backing for the idea.

With older children, it all becomes more complicated. Eczema can be associated with food allergy, so managing allergy is important, but food allergy does not necessarily exacerbate eczema. There may also be a link with nut and latex allergy, things like balloons and rubber gloves.

According to the NES, about 30 per cent of cases of childhood eczema could be triggered by food, but only about 10 per cent are triggered by food *alone*. As with other eczema triggers, it's not always easy to isolate the precise one which is causing a child's eczema to flare up. Dietary manipulation will not cure or even help eczema on its own so it's important to continue with a proper skincare regime.

Which foods may trigger eczema?

The answer is, almost any food can be a problem for a particular individual. However, the most common triggers are cow's milk and eggs. Soya, wheat, fish and nuts are also quite common causes of allergic reactions. If your eczema is affected by a food you may notice

- your skin becoming noticeably more itchy and uncomfortable, especially around your mouth, after eating it;
- an immediate food hypersensitivity reaction: you could develop a rash, redness or swelling of the skin anything from five minutes to two hours after eating the suspect food. You may have other symptoms too, up to and including the most serious kind of allergic reaction, known as anaphylaxis, which can lead to collapse and unconsciousness;
- a delayed hypersensitivity reaction – the most usual way for food to affect eczema – leading to a flare-up of your skin symptoms from 6 to 24 hours after eating the suspect food.

The only way to be absolutely sure which food has caused the problem is to keep a food diary, and/or to go on an 'exclusion diet'. This should really only be done under medical supervision, especially in the case of children. Everyone needs to eat a properly balanced and healthy diet which provides all the right nutrients for their age and lifestyle. Cutting out basic foods like cow's milk and wheat can cause all sorts of problems for growing children unless these staple items are replaced by others from the same food groups.

If you are fairly sure your child's eczema is diet-related, you should ask for a referral to a specialized paediatric dietician with special training in dietary manipulation for children.

An exclusion diet can be a complicated business. Usually the suspect food is removed from the diet for a period of anything from two to six weeks to see if the eczema symptoms improve.

Then a small amount of the food is reintroduced to see if the symptoms recur. As eczema may be affected by many different foodstuffs, working out exactly what the culprit is takes time and patience. It is also not always easy to persuade a child to give up foods he is especially fond of and possibly to eat others he doesn't like or hasn't tried before. It can also be difficult to cater for a family when one member is living on a restricted diet – and hard to explain to a child why he can't tuck into the foods his brothers and sisters are enjoying. So you do need commitment to take this route, although, of course, if it really does help the child's eczema it could be worth a try.

Nina, mum of 14-year-old Chelsea, found that the restricted diet an alternative health clinic prescribed for her daughter was helpful, but too strict for the then ten-year-old to stick to.

> She wasn't allowed anything tinned or processed, no sweets or chocolate, and no yeast. This last was the most difficult of all to give up as she was taking packed lunches to school at the time. Soda bread and some wraps don't contain yeast but I was amazed to find the stuff is practically everywhere!
>
> Chelsea tried this strict regime for about three months and there was a tremendous improvement in her skin, but she was also ten years old and just couldn't keep it up. She hated missing out on the treats her friends enjoyed.

There are alternatives to both cow's milk and wheat-based products – Allergy UK (for contact details see Useful addresses) has lots of information about these. Many supermarkets now sell their own 'free from ...' ranges, and their customer services departments can tell you which products are suitable for those unable to tolerate dairy products or wheat. However, the NES points out that children who can't tolerate cow's milk may also have a problem with both soya and goat's milk. The latter should not be given to babies under a year old anyway. Soya baby formula does contain the full range of nutrients necessary for growing children and can be found in health food shops.

Allergy testing

There are various tests available to find out just what causes allergic reactions – including eczema – in susceptible people. Skin-prick testing, and blood or RAST (radio allergosorbant) tests are among the most commonly used as they are clinically proven and pretty reliable. However, the results they give are not infallible, especially when relating to a small child.

Both kinds of tests can be done by your GP or practice nurse or in a hospital allergy clinic. Skin-prick testing involves putting a drop of allergen from the suspect food – wheat, milk, strawberries, citrus fruit, whatever – on the skin and then pricking it lightly. Within about fifteen minutes, the skin will become itchy and a raised weal appears if there is a positive reaction to that particular allergen. RAST testing involves taking a sample of blood and sending it away for laboratory analysis, with the results coming through in a couple of weeks. People with eczema are sometimes offered patch tests, where allergens are mixed with a substance such as Vaseline and spread on to special non-allergenic patches which then need to stay on the skin for 48 hours before any redness or swelling can be examined by a dermatologist.

Other types of testing such as hair analysis are sometimes advertised in the press or in alternative health clinics. Dermatologists point out that these tests have often not been clinically proven to work and they are not recommended.

Is it possible to prevent eczema?

If you have eczema yourself or if there are other atopic conditions such as asthma and hay fever in your family or your partner's, you might have asked yourself whether there is any way you can prevent your children developing these conditions, perhaps by changing your own diet during pregnancy or breast-feeding.

The evidence is inconclusive. According to both the NES and the British Association of Dermatologists, there is no proof at present that watching what you eat in pregnancy will make any difference to whether your baby develops eczema.

Your baby would be defined as at 'high risk' of developing eczema if both you and your partner and one or more siblings suffered from an atopic condition. If you are in that position, the NES recommends that you breast-feed your baby for at least six months and don't give her any solids before four months.

The *British Medical Journal* (*BMJ*) looked at the research around pregnant women's diets in 2006 and came to the conclusion that being careful what you eat during pregnancy doesn't prevent your baby developing eczema. The idea is that mums-to-be should avoid suspected allergens. One study looked at pregnant women and breast-feeding mothers who were avoiding milk, and another at women who were avoiding all dairy products, eggs, fish, beef or peanuts. In neither case did the change of diet have an effect on whether or not the babies developed eczema. The main difference the diets made was that mothers on a restricted diet had smaller babies. The *BMJ* is also not convinced that long-term breast-feeding of high-risk babies made them less likely to develop eczema.

Current advice on feeding 'high-risk' babies from the NES is that some solids, like baby rice, pureed fruits and vegetables and potatoes, should be given at six months, and that cow's milk, eggs, wheat and fish should be avoided. High-risk babies and small children should also not be given nuts or nut products like peanut butter.

Probiotics

Probiotics are the so-called 'friendly bacteria' that live in the gut, helping us to digest our food and destroying other, harmful bacteria. Probiotics exist naturally in some foods and can be added to foods and drinks such as yoghurt, milk and soya drinks. They are also available as supplements.

Sian, mum of seven-year-old Simon, found that giving him probiotic supplements as suggested by her local allergy clinic improved the condition of his skin. Articles by Finnish researchers in the medical journal *The Lancet* in 2001 and 2003 describe clinical trials of a probiotic supplement called *lactobacillus GG*, which was given to women in the final month of pregnancy and then to their babies. The researchers found that these supplements did seem to reduce the incidence of eczema in babies and small children. At two years old, 23 per cent of the babies who were given probiotics had developed eczema, compared with 46 per cent of the babies who had been given a placebo. At four years old, 25 per cent of the 'probiotic' babies had eczema, compared with 50 per cent of the 'placebo' babies.

More research is needed to see whether this treatment is definitely to be recommended to pregnant women in high-risk families. It is thought that probiotics might help the baby's immune system to develop properly and prevent allergic conditions such as eczema developing.

What else might help?

Dietician Emma Mills has some key recommendations for a 'healthy skin' diet:

- Choose spreading fats and cooking oils which contain more Omega–3 than Omega–6 fat, such as butter, olive oil, rapeseed oil, walnut oil or linseed or flaxseed oil. You can mix half butter and half oil together in a food processor to make a spread, and use walnut or linseed or flaxseed oil to make salad dressings.
- Eat more fish and seafood and less meat. Try to eat three portions of fish a week, with at least one of them being an oily

fish such as salmon, fresh tuna, trout, mackerel, sardines or herring.
- Eat plenty of green, leafy vegetables, such as rocket, watercress, spinach, fresh basil and coriander, in soups, sandwiches, salads, sauces and marinades.
- Eat at least five portions of fruit and vegetables per day, including highly coloured varieties. Make soups and smoothies as well as eating them raw or lightly cooked.
- Drink at least eight glasses of plain water every day. Skin needs to be hydrated to function properly and water aids the healing of sore, inflamed skin.

More about essential fatty acids

Essential fatty acids like Omega–6 and Omega–3 are so-called because they are essential for our well-being. Our bodies cannot make them themselves, so we have to obtain them from our diets. Briefly, they are converted within the body into 'longer chain fats', each of which has a definite function. The Omega–3 fat, EPA or eicosapentaenoic acid, is used to make something called leukotriene B5 which seems to have an anti-inflammatory effect. If you replace some of the Omega–6 fat with Omega–3, you might be able to alter your body's immune response and this could have an effect on your eczema. Dietician Emma Mills advises people with eczema to try an Omega–3 fatty acid supplement in addition to the healthy eating guidelines mentioned above, especially if they don't like eating fish or seafood.

Charlotte Vohtz, founder of the Green People health and beauty company, also recommends a diet enriched with Omega–3 essential fatty acids to improve the condition of problem skin. As we have already seen, she started the company because her young daughter had severe eczema, which cleared up under this regime.

At first glance, the fat and oil content of my daughter's diet seemed very good, with plenty of vegetable oils and few animal fats. I thought that this would make sure she was getting enough essential fatty acids.

However, the more I studied this area, the more I came to see that while her diet was providing plenty of Omega–6 fatty acids, it was actually very low in Omega–3 fatty acids. Like most Western diets, this was providing a ratio between Omega–6 and Omega–3 of around 25:1. Looking at the body's requirements, I found that the ideal ratio was closer to 4:1.

By adding a supplement to Sandra's diet providing Omega–6 and Omega–3 fatty acids in a ratio of 1:3, that is three times as much Omega–3 as Omega–6, we were able to correct the imbalance and restore the ideal levels needed for a healthy body.

Margaret Weeds, founder of organic health and beauty company Essential Care, based in Suffolk, also found that a change of diet benefited her children's skin.

I began formulating our products twenty years ago, motivated by the lack of wholesome remedies suitable for my own and my family's eczema-prone, sensitive skin.

My youngest daughter had both asthma and eczema and I wondered if it was caused by her school meals. I changed her over to packed lunches and her skin improved at once. It seemed to be processed food full of chemical additives that affected her. I could always tell if she had eaten flavoured crisps from someone else's lunch box! You have to live in the real world, though. It can be hard for children to go to a party and have to ask for a glass of water rather than a fizzy drink. Though there are healthier alternatives available now than when my daughter was young.

I also recommend essential fatty acid supplements such as those in evening primrose or starflower (borage) oil. It seems that some people with eczema don't have the ability to break down fatty acids into components the body can use.

As is so often the case with eczema, the people I spoke to for the book recommended a variety of diet changes. Eggs, oranges and tomatoes were mentioned as possible triggers. Some said that what they ate seemed to make little difference. Others recommended evening primrose oil capsules and aloe vera capsules.

Anne, who is 63 and has had eczema for most of her life, says,

I have had food allergies for the past twenty-five years and it's only in the last five that I have come to understand that I seem to have an excess of acid in my digestive system. I can't eat most grains, dairy products, lactose, artificial sweeteners, some meats, some vegetables, almost all fresh and dried fruits, oils and nuts – it's almost easier to say what I *can* eat. However, I have learned to cope and have been told on one of my very few visits to the doctor that I am as healthy as a horse!

8

Complementary therapies

If you are living with a chronic condition like eczema, for which there's no current cure, it's always tempting to take a look at what complementary therapies have to offer. Some people don't need to, of course, because existing mainstream treatments like emollients and steroids seem to suit their skin and are effective in dealing with any flare-ups. But if you don't find them helpful, or if you like the idea of choosing a gentler, more 'natural' kind of treatment that doesn't have the possible side-effects of steroids, you might wonder if complementary therapies could help you. There are so many possible treatments, though, some pretty much accepted by everyone but the most die-hard sceptics, some sounding frankly dippy. How do you choose?

Almost all those with eczema I spoke to for this book had experimented with various kinds of 'alternative' treatments, ranging from herbal lotions and potions to acupuncture – with varying degrees of success. Even dietary manipulation and the use of essential fatty acid supplements, discussed in the last chapter, seem to lie somewhere on the border between officially sanctioned, conventional medical practice and the alternatives.

Many doctors today understand the value of complementary therapies; some will refer people to reputable 'alternative' practitioners. Homoeopathic treatments are sometimes available on the NHS, either from specially trained GPs or at one of the five NHS homoeopathic hospitals – the Royal London, Liverpool Mossley Hill, Glasgow, Bristol and Tunbridge Wells. There has been considerable interest also in what traditional Chinese medicine can offer in the way of treatments for eczema and other skin conditions.

However, it's important to strike a note of caution. Dermatologist Sue Lewis-Jones from Ninewells Hospital in Dundee says,

> There is no evidence for most complementary medicine and buying on the Internet can be very risky. I have heard of patients obtaining products and being quite unaware they contained potent steroids. Western drugs are well-researched and contain one ingredient only, while in plants there may be several ingredients. Chinese herbs do work but do not seem to be entirely safe and there have been some deaths after using them. Long-term side-effects are also not known.

The National Eczema Society points out that complementary medicine is not a cure for eczema. However, they say that many people do use complementary treatments to reduce the impact of eczema on their quality of life. These therapies can also be useful in helping people to relax, to relieve stress and to control symptoms, therefore possibly reducing the need for steroid creams and ointments.

It is often easy for the unscrupulous, or downright cranky, to prey on the vulnerabilities of people desperate to find a 'miracle cure' for a troublesome condition like eczema. Complementary therapies can and do help some people, but if you are considering going along that route there are a few points you have to remember:

- Many complementary therapies have not been subjected to the rigorous scientific, double-blind, placebo-controlled clinical trials that pharmaceutical drugs have to go through before they are allowed on the market. When trials do take place, the results are often inconclusive or disappointing.
- Not everything that is 'natural' is harmless. There are many natural allergens and poisons, as well as complementary therapies which react with other drugs you may be taking.

- You should always find a therapist through one of the accredited bodies which regulate their work such as the Acupuncture Council or the National Institute of Medical Herbalists.
- Be very sceptical about anyone who claims to be able to offer a miracle cure.
- Check out premises – which should be scrupulously clean, bright and well lit – practitioners' qualifications and the general ambiance of the place before parting with your money.
- Always tell your GP or skin specialist that you are trying, or thinking of trying, any kind of 'alternative' treatment. Don't stop using your conventional treatments.
- The National Eczema Society always has up-to-date information about complementary treatments.

Having said all that, some complementary treatments can work very well for eczema and other skin problems.

Herbal medicine

At one time, all medicine was 'herbal medicine'. Much of modern medicine is descended from the old herbal concoctions brewed up by the 'wise women' of the past. They had learned by long years of trial and error that willow bark, for example, had pain-relieving properties. We now know that was because it contained a substance related to aspirin. Some of the modern drugs used in the treatment of cancer are derived from a kind of periwinkle, and of course morphine comes from the opium poppy. It isn't surprising that herbal remedies can be useful in the treatment of eczema.

Trudy Norris of the National Institute of Medical Herbalists says,

> We do see a lot of patients with eczema and other chronic skin problems, both children and adults. Either they have not found another treatment that works, or they might be wary of using steroids.

When someone comes to me I will take a detailed health history. Sometimes dietary factors are involved, sometimes not. I look at their skin in detail and sometimes prescribe herbs that influence the lymphatic system, herbs that affect the circulation, the adrenal glands, or sometimes the nervous system.

Any prescribing is done on a individual basis. A patient could be eating the wrong diet, be very stressed, have low blood pressure or a significant digestive problem, as well as eczema. Typically I will prescribe a mixture of between four and six different herbs. There is no *one* herb which cures eczema. I might make dietary recommendations as well.

There are also topical treatments. Creams based on comfrey or calendula can be very effective. I would never promise a complete cure but we can help many people. Several visits will be necessary, depending on the severity of the eczema. I refine the treatment as we go along, but it is always based on individual need. Herbalists acknowledge the fact that every patient is different and so is their eczema.

Trudy also points out that over-the-counter herbal preparations such as calendula cream may be effective for someone who has occasional brief flare-ups, but that anyone with severe eczema should consult a qualified practitioner.

Preparations containing liquorice root, burdock root and sarsaparilla have also been used as traditional treatments for eczema.

Homoeopathy

Homoeopathy is one of the most popular forms of complementary medicine but it is often misunderstood, or confused with herbal medicine. Like herbal medicine, it is tailored to the individual, so that one person's prescription will not necessarily be the same as the next person's, even though they both have eczema. This is because homoeopathy works holistically, which is to say it treats the whole person, not just the disease. A homoeopathic consultation takes much longer than a visit to the average GP, and the homoeopath or homoeopathic doctor (there is a difference!) will want to know as much as possible about the individual and the illness before she prescribes.

There is a specialist skin clinic at the Royal London Homoeopathic Hospital (RLHH), which treats eczema and dermatitis in addition to other skin conditions. In a 1997 survey of 500 patients, 68 per cent reported an improvement in their skin and about two-thirds found that they could reduce or stop using conventional medication after attending the RLHH.

The basic principle of homoeopathy is that 'like cures like'. In other words, an illness is treated with a substance which in a healthy person produces similar symptoms to those displayed by the patient. The idea is not so much to suppress the symptoms, but to trigger the body's own healing processes.

As with herbal medicines, you can buy homoeopathic remedies over the counter, but unlike conventional medication, you need to match them to the individual, not just the symptoms. Homoeopathic remedies for eczema might include:

- Arsen. alb: for dry, very flaky skin which 'burns' when it has been scratched. It is worse in winter and improved by warm weather or a warm bath. The patient is anxious and a worrier; the intelligent, fastidious, precise type.
- Graphites: for eczema mostly found in the skin folds. Skin is cracked and may ooze liquid. Nails may be ridged or thickened. Women may find their eczema is worse pre-menstrually. The patient often feels chilly and is weepy, indecisive and cautious.
- Sulphur: for extremely itchy, burning skin which bleeds when scratched. Heat makes it worse. The patient is aggressive and argumentative and rarely feels the cold.

Of course, a trained homoeopath will be able to prescribe much more precisely. Dr Peter Fisher, MRCP, FFHom, who is the consultant skin specialist at the Royal London Homoeopathic Hospital, told the NES that his clinic could do something for most people with eczema and that the results are particularly noticeable in children.

> Homoeopathy works quite slowly in long-standing cases. We sometimes say 'a month's treatment for every year you have had it'. Generally, you should not stop other treatments suddenly when starting homoeopathy. I usually advise a gradual reduction in steroid creams once improvement has started.

Like medical herbalist Trudy Norris, Dr Fisher recommends calendula cream as skin symptoms improve.

As with all complementary practitioners, you should make sure any homoeopath you consult is properly qualified. Some, like Dr Fisher, are medical doctors who have done the usual medical training before specializing in homoeopathy. In addition to their medical degree they have the letters 'MFHom' or 'FFHom' after their names. Others are not medically trained, but those registered with the Society of Homoeopaths have 'RSHom' after their names. Contact the British Homoeopathic Association (see Useful addresses) for information about practitioners in your area.

Traditional Chinese medicine

Traditional Chinese medicine or TCM is a 5,000-year-old medical system based on totally different principles from those of conventional or Western medicine. Chinese doctors believe that health and well-being depend on the correct flow of the life-force or chi through the body, which is channelled along 12 'meridians' or pathways, six of them being 'Yin' (feminine, cold, passive) and six 'Yang' (masculine, hot, active). Chinese medicine is aimed at balancing these two elements.

Two of the most common Chinese treatments are acupuncture, accepted by many Western doctors as a useful form of pain relief, and Chinese herbal medicine. Some people with eczema find acupuncture helpful: this involves the insertion of extremely fine needles at appropriate points on the body. Other, related forms of treatment are available for those who find it difficult to tolerate needles.

In the early 1990s a group of children with very severe eczema took part in a scientifically conducted trial at Great Ormond Street Hospital in London, in which they were given a herbal tea specially formulated by a recognized Chinese practitioner.

The children who had been given the herbal tea experienced a quite dramatic improvement in the condition of their skin compared with those given a placebo. The results were later replicated in adults and initially it looked as though Chinese herbal medicine was going to offer the best hope of a 'cure' for eczema. However, the National Eczema Society urged caution and called for more research, pointing out that

- this treatment didn't work for everyone and was trialled on a specially selected group;
- it was not known exactly how the treatment worked or what long-term side-effects there might be;
- there have been reports of liver damage in some people using Chinese herbal medicine;
- Chinese medicinal plants are not licensed for use here and it is difficult to know exactly what is being prescribed;
- in 1999 the *BMJ* reported that 8 out of 11 creams recommended by Chinese herbalists actually contained steroids, although those prescribed them were not informed of this.

Anyone thinking of consulting a Chinese medical practitioner for eczema treatment is advised to inform their own GP and dermatologist and to check the qualifications of anyone they consult very carefully.

AcuMedic (for contact details see Useful addresses) is the largest Chinese medical organization outside Asia with branches in London and Bath. Their doctors are fully qualified in both Chinese and Western medicine and follow the code of practice of their own Chinese Medical Institute and Register. They say that between 70 and 80 per cent of those who come to them with eczema can be helped.

'Chinese medicine is based on syndromes, not just on symptoms,' explained their spokeswoman.

> All treatments are tailored to the individual because Chinese medicine believes that a condition like eczema can be associated with the functioning of the lungs, stomach, the heart or the blood, the reasons being different in different patients. A Chinese doctor will ask about your general health, not only your skin, and will look at your tongue and take your pulse before making a diagnosis. We use only premium-quality herbs and no animal products.

Juliet, 30, had tried every kind of treatment, both conventional and complementary, before a friend recommended Chinese medicine to her.

> I was prescribed an eight-week course of acupuncture, plus a herbal infusion I had to boil up and drink every day, and assorted herbal creams. The herbal infusion looked and tasted absolutely awful. After a week, my skin was no better and I felt like giving up but the Chinese doctors persuaded me to continue with the treatment. Slowly, my skin began to improve until the dryness and flakiness disappeared. Sometimes I have no eczema at all now. I still take Chinese herbal capsules and use their skin cream and I feel, and look, like a different person.

Avene spring water

The Avene Dermatological Spa, situated high in the mountains of south-western France, has been treating skin problems since the eighteenth century. Treatments are based on the use of pure local spring water, which contains a particular level of minerals, trace elements and other constituents that seem to benefit skin conditions like eczema. Each person is given a specially devised, individual treatment plan which can include baths in running spring water, showers and spraying. Rest, massage, wet-wrapping and sunbathing as well as drinking approximately a litre and a half of spring water per day may also be prescribed as part of the treatment. The spa can treat children as well as adults.

Like many complementary treatments, it can sound far-fetched, but results are often very good, as Elizabeth, who has visited the spa twice with her teenage daughter, says.

> I have chronic eczema which is effectively a disability. Jade's eczema is just on her feet so isn't as obvious.
>
> I've been treated at the dermatology department of my local hospital and also at the Royal London Homoeopathic Hospital. My skin has been damaged by steroids so I am especially interested in complementary treatments.
>
> Our two weeks at Avene benefited both of us. We had individual treatment packages. In my case this involved underwater massage, wraps with their own Avene creams, and attending a one-and-a-half-hour anti-scratching workshop where we learned different techniques to help us break the itch–scratch cycle. Being there was a complete experience. It is such a beautiful place and you are so well cared for, seeing a doctor every three days. My eczema is stress-related, but I was able to relax completely in a healing environment. They don't claim a 'cure' but they help you to manage your skin condition and emphasize the importance of a balanced diet, plenty of water to drink and plenty of rest.
>
> When I returned home I continued to use Avene skincare products because they worked for my skin better than any others I have tried.

Dead Sea mud

The Dead Sea, with its hot sunny climate, is situated about 1,300 ft (396 m) below sea level in between Israel and Jordan, and has been recognized for its therapeutic properties since ancient times. Bathing in the world's saltiest lake is said to benefit skin conditions (notably psoriasis) as well as other health problems like arthritis. Mud from the Dead Sea contains high levels of mineral salts which are said to help skin conditions, and products made from refined Dead Sea mud may have healing properties, though there is little research evidence for their effect on eczema.

Hypnotherapy

Hypnotherapy as a treatment for eczema has become more and more accepted by mainstream medicine. There is scientific evidence to suggest that it is not just helpful in reducing the stress and anxiety which can cause eczema flare-ups, but that it even has a measurable effect on the functioning of the immune system.

Dr Ann Williamson is a former GP who has treated many people who had eczema. She currently works as a hypnotherapist.

> I have used hypnosis to help eczema patients since the early 1990s. When I was running a simple, three-session stress and anxiety management group, on several occasions patients would come up to me after the second session and tell me that their eczema had markedly improved. I also treated patients at a local dermatology department, with good results.

Hypnotherapy is often confused with the 'stage' version where members of the audience are persuaded to make idiots of themselves for entertainment, but it can also be a useful therapeutic tool. Hypnosis is not sleep or brain-washing, it's simply a dreamy state, induced either by yourself or by a trained therapist, which is associated with profound relaxation. Ann Williamson uses 'goal-directed imagery' to help her eczema patients.

> I use a classic image which is cool, calm and comfortable. My patients are asked to imagine themselves walking into a healing pool or smoothing on a healing cream, and to 'see' their skin looking the way they want it to look. The skin and the mind are closely linked and most people's eczema is made worse by stress. I think at least a fifth of patients are able to use the techniques to help control the inflammatory response in their skin disease. Others can help themselves to feel less troubled by their symptoms, and maybe interrupt the itch–scratch cycle.

Of course, it is vital when consulting a hypnotherapist to make sure that he or she is properly qualified and a member of the British Society of Experimental and Clinical Hypnosis or the

British Society of Medical and Dental Hypnosis (for contact details see Useful addresses).

Aloe vera

The aloe vera plant is a succulent, related to lilies, onions, garlic and asparagus. It grows in warm, dry climates and has been used for its therapeutic properties for 4,000 years. Gels and creams containing aloe vera can be used on the skin and aloe vera drinks can also have healing properties.

Dr Peter Atherton was a GP for more than thirty years. He always had a special interest in dermatology and was impressed when an eczema patient showed him the improvement in her skin after using an aloe vera cream.

> No-one had heard of it at that time but when I researched aloe vera, I discovered it had been used for healing damaged skin since the days of Hippocrates. I studied it for two years and then wrote my book, *The Essential Aloe Vera*, which looked at all the world-wide research.
>
> It isn't myth or magic, it's medicine. Drinking aloe vera gel can provide the body with micronutrients missing from our modern diets. It works as an immunomodulator on conditions related to an unbalanced immune system, such as eczema. It has a slight anti-histamine effect. It can reduce itching and inflammation and quieten down the skin. I would not say it offers a permanent cure for eczema but it does suppress the troublesome symptoms.

Aloe vera is still seen as an 'alternative' treatment for eczema, though Dr Atherton says it is being used in a pilot study on children with severe skin disease at Great Ormond Street Hospital.

More relaxation techniques

You will have noticed that many complementary practitioners mention that their treatments work holistically, dealing with the whole body and the whole person rather than just the eczema symptoms. If your eczema flare-ups tend to come at times when you are especially stressed, you could benefit from any kind of relaxation technique that appeals to you, from yoga to aromatherapy (though you should be careful not to use any essential oils which could cause an allergic reaction on sore, inflamed skin), shiatsu, reflexology, creative visualization or simply listening to one of the many relaxation CDs which are readily available.

Yoga

Yoga, for example, has been developed over thousands of years to promote good physical health and inner peace. The word 'yoga' comes from a Sanskrit word meaning 'union' and yoga is designed to promote union between mind and body by the use of correct breathing, physical exercises and meditation. You don't have to be a contortionist and the best way to learn is to join a class.

Bach flower remedies

Dr Edward Bach was a homoeopath who devised 38 special 'flower remedies' to be used for particular personalities and particular emotional states. Bach Rescue Remedy, widely available from health food stores and specialist pharmacies, is a composite of five flower remedies and is specially recommended for everyday stress and emotional crises.

Meditation

Different kinds of meditation – transcendental meditation or Buddhist meditation among them – can help those who practise them achieve a state of deep relaxation. Once you have been taught to meditate, 20 minutes twice a day can benefit conditions such as irritable bowel syndrome (IBS) and asthma as well as anxiety and high blood pressure. EEGs (electroencephalograms) have shown that meditation produces alpha-waves in the brain, associated with rest and relaxation.

Autogenic training (AT)

Devised by a German psychiatrist and neurologist in the 1920s, AT is similar to meditation and self-hypnosis and helps people to switch off the sympathetic *fight-or-flight* nervous system which over-reacts in times of stress. Learning simple relaxation techniques can allow the parasympathetic *rest, relaxation and recreation* nervous system to come into play instead.

AT was introduced into the UK in the 1970s but is still less widely known than other methods of relaxation like yoga or transcendental meditation. According to the British Autogenic Society, an individual learns to experience a state called passive concentration which enables him or her to break through the vicious circle of excessive stress.

You don't need special clothing to learn AT and no athletic poses are required. Most courses consist of a series of six or eight 90-minute or two-hour sessions, held weekly, and reinforced by exercises to practise at home. AT can be used to benefit almost anyone and can help with both physical and emotional difficulties caused or exacerbated by stress and tension; it has been scientifically proved to help stress-related conditions including high blood pressure.

As well as benefiting those suffering from skin problems, it can also be useful for anxiety, panic attacks, irritable bowel syndrome, sleep disorders, tension headaches, arthritis, asthma, PMT and urinary problems.

T'ai chi

This is a combination of gentle martial art, exercise and meditation. Like most Chinese therapies, it's aimed at balancing the body's chi, or vital force, and promoting harmony and calm. 'Meditation in motion' is one description of this ancient art, which is now very popular in the UK.

Reflexology

Reflexology operates on the proposition that the body is divided into ten different energy zones. Each channel relates to a particular bodily zone, and to the organs in that zone. By applying pressure to the appropriate terminal in the form of a small, specialized massage, a practitioner can determine which energy pathways are blocked.

Experts claim that all the organs of the body are reflected in the feet. They also believe that reflexology aids the removal of waste products and blockages within the energy channels, improving circulation and gland function. Many people do find reflexology very relaxing, and as well as reducing stress it can improve depression.

Reflexologists also believe that reflexology improves the general elasticity of the skin because it stimulates the whole circulation system, improving the transport of oxygen, nutrients and other necessary chemical messengers round the body, and so improving the general tone and quality of the skin.

Acupuncture

This involves inserting fine needles at energy channels (meridians) in the body which are believed to correspond with certain internal organs. It can be a highly specialized process – it is thought there are as many as 2,000 acupuncture points on the body. The needles are believed to increase, decrease or unblock the flow of chi energy, disturbance of which is thought to lead to illness. Acupuncture is often used to relieve stress-related health problems, and research shows it can also be effective as a means of pain relief.

It is thought to be safe in properly trained hands but should be avoided in the first three months of pregnancy.

Shiatsu

Shiatsu has been compared with acupuncture, except that it avoids the stress of needles piercing your skin. Whereas acupuncture concentrates on specific points along the meridians or energy channels, shiatsu focuses on the meridians that link the points. These meridians are believed to contain the chi energy, which, when blocked, may manifest as ill health. Shiatsu is believed to remove such blockages.

In shiatsu, the practitioner uses his or her hands, elbows, knees and feet instead of needles, and the treatment involves gentle stretching, holding and applying pressure to the client's body. As a result, the energy flow is stimulated, as is blood circulation. There is generally also increased flexibility and improved posture. People who use shiatsu commonly report feeling much more relaxed afterwards.

9

What about the future?

Research into eczema is ongoing, but as it is such a complex condition involving so many different factors, both genetic and environmental, it doesn't look as though a 'cure' is likely to emerge in the foreseeable future. Most research seems to be in the area of management, helping to make the lives of those with eczema easier.

For example, some recent research at the University of Nottingham Centre for Evidence-Based Dermatology, reported in the medical journal *The Lancet*, discovered that eczema in children was 56 per cent more prevalent in hard-water areas. The theory is that either the mineral salts in hard water lead to more dry, irritated skin, or possibly families in hard-water areas are forced to use more soap, drying out their children's skin in the process. Further experiments are being carried out using specially installed water-softeners in 310 selected families to see what kind of impact that has on children's eczema. The study is due to report its findings in 2009 or 2010.

Another researcher in the same department is looking at how environmental factors affect eczema flare-ups. Children in this study are asked to wear special monitoring equipment which measures things like heat and humidity. The impact of gut parasites, which might protect people against the development of atopic conditions, is also being looked at, and of course this links into the use of probiotic supplements to prevent eczema developing, as mentioned in Chapter 7.

Recent years have seen some interesting developments and hopeful signs. In early 2006, the British Skin Foundation announced that one of its research projects, at the University of Dundee, had achieved a real breakthrough when they managed to identify the gene which causes dry skin. This gene produces a protein called filaggrin, which helps the skin to form its protective outer barrier, and its discovery could lead to more effective therapies being produced which might actually tackle the root cause of eczema rather than just treating the symptoms. As Professor Irwin McLean, Professor of Human Genetics at Dundee University and leader of the research team, says, 'If you imagine eczema as a burning building, up till now we have just been throwing buckets of water on to the roof. Now that we know where the problem is, we may be able to produce more effective therapies.'

Professor McLean has been working on genetic skin diseases for fifteen years, with most of his work concentrating on tracking down the faulty genes responsible for them.

> One of the most common is something called ichthyosis vulgaris, a scaly skin condition which affects about one in 250 children. We identified the gene for that a year ago. In the process of investigating it we realized that many children with it get eczema too. It turned out that both conditions are caused by the same thing, a faulty gene which is carried by about 10 per cent of the European population.
>
> This gene is located on chromosome No. 1, which is a susceptibility region for eczema, and produces the protein filaggrin. In normal skin this protein is abundant in the outer layers of the epidermis, which is made up of dead skin cells chemically modified to act a bit like clingfilm and stop the skin drying out. So, we have discovered that about 10 per cent of the population only produce about half the amount of filaggrin they need and some people don't make any at all, which is why they get severe eczema.
>
> The second function of the epidermis, in addition to stopping moisture loss, is to stop chemicals, pathogens, allergens and foreign bodies generally getting into the body. Without the right amount of filaggrin all this junk *does* get in. The body's immune system reacts to it and the skin becomes inflamed.

There have been two main theories about the causes of eczema. One concerns an over-active immune system, and the second is that there is something wrong with the barrier function of the skin. Most of the research which has been done over the past twenty years has been into the immune system, but our research suggests that a problem with the skin's barrier function may actually be more important.

Since Professor McLean's prize-winning research findings were published in 2006 there have been 25 further studies confirming his results. It is still early days but the implications for those with eczema could be that new kinds of treatments could be developed.

As Professor McLean explains,

Until now, most of the available treatments have been aimed at dampening down the immune system response. In future, perhaps we should be looking at drugs or other treatments which increase the barrier function of the skin. Of course, emollients already do that to a degree.

We need to develop new drugs which boost the gene to produce more filaggrin. If we could increase the gene's activity by about 50 per cent, that might be enough, and we are already working on drugs to do that. There is also the possibility that existing drugs might have this effect, which would speed up treatment, as the normal development time for new drugs can be as much as ten years.

We estimate that people who are carriers of this faulty gene have about a 60 per cent chance of developing eczema. We are also looking at the other 40 per cent to see if we can discover anything special about their genetic make-up or their environment. If we could modify the environment for people at risk we might be able to prevent them developing eczema. Now we have found the gene it will be easy to test those who are at risk and I'm confident that new methods of prevention and treatment will emerge.

Professor McLean's findings about filaggrin have already been factored into the research which is being done in Nottingham on the effects of water-softeners.

As with so many diseases, it looks as though research into eczema is proceeding in small steps rather than with one major life-changing breakthrough. In early 2006, doctors at Newcastle University reported the results of a randomized clinical trial of a 40-year-old immunosuppressant drug called azathioprine as a treatment for eczema. Like many drugs of this type it is very strong, with some undesirable possible side-effects, but the research team have found a way of tailoring the dose to suit the individual and minimize these problems.

Originally developed in the 1960s to treat kidney transplant patients and prevent rejection of their new organs, azathioprine has also been used to treat auto-immune conditions like rheumatoid arthritis and lupus as well as childhood leukaemia.

Professor Nick Reynolds of Newcastle University:

We have been working on this since about 2000. The results of our first trials were promising so we set up a formal, placebo-controlled trial with the help of 63 adults with eczema, who all had moderate to severe disease which had not responded to existing treatments.

It was important to prove that the effect was more than just placebo as it is already known that the whole process of being monitored tends to improve patients' eczema anyway! Perhaps the fact that the patients feel 'special' helps them to comply better with their treatment, but in any event we needed to see whether azathioprine actually worked.

Because it is a drug that has been used for some time quite a lot is already known about how it works. We know that an individual's response to the drug is affected by the amount of a particular enzyme they have in their body. The enzyme is called TPMT and about one in 200 people don't have any of it in their bodies at all – in which case, the drug is too dangerous for them to use. About 20 per cent of the population metabolize the drug slowly, and need an adjusted dose. Because we knew all this we were able to give all our patients a dose of the drug which was individually tailored for them. We found it was very effective, and because they had had an individualized dose, side-effects were minimized.

The trial, which was funded by the British Skin Foundation, found that azathioprine was indeed an effective treatment for eczema. The effects also seemed to be quite long-lasting, giving several months of relatively problem-free skin.

The idea of testing people's individual responses to particular drugs and tailoring the dosage accordingly seems a promising one, and not only for azathioprine. It may also have implications for other drugs, and indeed other treatments, in the future. Professor Reynolds says that this area, known as 'pharmaco-genetics', seems a promising field of study for future research. Like Professor McLean, he thinks that in future more attention will be paid to researching the problems around the barrier function of the skin, rather than researchers concentrating on the problems with the immune system which may cause eczema.

'If your skin is leaky, more allergens get in!' he says. 'Once patients realize that, they can see the logic behind applying lots of emollient. Researchers are actively gene-hunting at the moment.'

Useful addresses

The huge rise in the incidence of allergic conditions like eczema in the last thirty years has meant that the whole subject has hit the headlines on several occasions – which is good news for those battling to deal with eczema on a day-to-day basis. As often happens in the National Health Service, treatment facilities tend to depend on where you live. Dermatology is not a glamorous speciality for doctors and it takes up a very small part of GPs' training.

Looking at eczema as part of the increasing problem of allergies, it's obvious that there is a need for more specialist services. The Royal College of Physicians' report *Allergy – The Unmet Need*, published in 2003, pointed out that there are only six full-time specialist allergy clinics in the UK and that they are concentrated in the south-east of the country. More funds are needed for treatment centres as well as research. In 2004, a five-year European-wide research programme was set up, co-ordinated by Paul van Cauwenberge, Dean of the medical faculty at the University of Ghent in Belgium, and involving 25 different universities and research institutes over the whole continent. It's not only in Britain that allergies are becoming more prevalent. Researchers are hoping that some of their work will provide answers to the questions which still puzzle allergists and dermatologists – just what is it about the way we live today that has caused the two- to three-fold rise in conditions like eczema in the last twenty years?

In the meantime, while we wait for a scientific breakthrough, there are organizations, charities, campaigning groups and commercial companies helping to make life a little easier for those living with eczema. Whether you are looking for information about the emollient you have been prescribed, a source of pure cotton or silk clothing for yourself or your child, or a reputable complementary practitioner, the contact details listed below should be able to help you.

Organizations

Allergy UK
3 White Oak Square
London Road
Swanley
Kent BR8 7AG
Helpline: 01322 619898
Website: www.allergyuk.org

An excellent source of help and advice on all forms of allergic illness including eczema.

Asthma UK
Summit House
70 Wilson Street
London EC2A 2DB
Tel.: 020 7786 5000
Advice Line: 08457 01 02 03 (9 a.m. to 5 p.m., Monday to Friday)
Website: www.asthma.org.uk

Gives information on Kick Asthma Holidays, aimed at children and teens, and suitable for those with eczema and other allergic conditions as well as asthma.

British Association of Dermatologists
Website: www.bad.org.uk

Provides patient information leaflets and very useful information about general skincare topics.

British Skin Foundation
4 Fitzroy Square
London W1T 5HQ
Tel.: 020 7391 6341
Website: www.britishskinfoundation.org.uk

This organization concentrates on research and fundraising, and also provides information for patients.

National Eczema Society (NES)
Hill House
Highgate Hill
London N19 5NA
Helpline: 0870 241 3604 (8 a.m. to 8 p.m., Monday to Friday)
Website: www.eczema.org

A membership organization offering support, information and guidance for those with eczema and their families, the NES publishes a quarterly journal, *Exchange*, and has a full list of factsheets on eczema-related topics.

Clothing and bedding

AllergyBestBuys
Hill Top Farm
Heights Lane
Bingley BD16 3AF

Tel.: 08707 455002
Website: www.allergybestbuys.co.uk

Suppliers of eczema and asthma allergy products such as duvets, sheets, pillows, clothing and other items for the home, including 'Medivac' and 'Medivap' specialist vacuum cleaners. They provide a catalogue for online shopping and ordering by post.

www.eparenting.co.uk

A parenting website that includes a list of retailers selling pure and organic cotton clothing, plus a second list of companies which sell clothing specifically for eczema sufferers.

Greenfibres
99 High Street
Totnes
Devon TQ9 5PF
Tel.: 01803 868001
Website: www.greenfibres.com

A company selling bedding and skin-friendly clothing; personal callers to the shop are welcome from 10 a.m. to 5 p.m., Monday to Saturday; an online catalogue and shop is also available.

Healthy House
The Old Co-op
Lower Street
Ruscombe
Stroud GL6 6BU
Tel.: 01453 752216
Lower Rate Call: 0845 450 5950
Website: www.healthy-house.co.uk

Provides a catalogue containing pretty much all you need to make major lifestyle changes to improve your skin condition. They sell dust mite-proof bedding including mattress protectors, pillow and duvet covers and organic cotton clothes for children, as well as Ecos organic paints and other DIY items.

John Lewis and other department stores sell anti-allergy bedding.

Pure Cotton Comfort
PO Box 71
Carnforth LA5 9YA
Tel.: 01524 730093
Website: www.eczemaclothing.com

A company started by a mother who could not find suitable clothing for her severely allergic child; its range now includes mitten T-shirts, babygros, pyjamas, sheet sleeping bags, socks, tights and schoolwear for children, plus underwear and nightwear for adults, as well as a small range of toiletries.

Tower Health Ltd
Unit 17
Wilford Business and Industrial Park
Ruddington Lane
Nottingham NG11 7EP
Tel.: 08450 066 077
Website: www.tower-health.co.uk

Sells a variety of anti-allergy products including mattress covers and pillows.

Skin-friendly toiletries

The rise in the incidence of eczema and other allergic conditions has led to a corresponding rise in the number of companies offering skin-friendly and hypo-allergenic products, ranging from major cosmetic companies to small one-woman operations. The British Skin Foundation does not recommend the use of so-called 'natural' or 'herbal' products, but some users do find they can use them without problems.

It should always be borne in mind that the fact that any product – cosmetic or household – is labelled 'natural' does not mean that your individual skin will not react badly to it. As those dealing with eczema on an everyday basis know, almost any product may cause a flare-up. Trial and error can also be an expensive way of finding out what does and doesn't suit your skin. However, at present it seems to be the only way.

Essential Care
Tel.: 01638 716593
Website: www.essential-care.co.uk

A small company founded by a mother to cater for her own family's sensitive skin.

Grandma Vine's
Tel.: 01455 556281
Website: www.grandma-vines.co.uk

Produces a range of skin-friendly toiletries created specially for people suffering from eczema, dermatitis and very dry skin.

Green People
Tel.: 01403 740350
Website: www.greenpeople.co.uk

A company started by a mother in order to make products suitable for her young daughter's sensitive skin. The range now includes more than a hundred items, from deodorant to baby skin care and supplements.

Hope's Relief Cream
Tel.: 0845 094 0402
Website: www.beautynaturals.com

Devised by an Australian naturopath, Jacqueline Hope, and only available by mail order and on the Internet, this product did well in a *Guardian* reader survey.

Jurlique
Tel.: 08707 700980
Website: www.jurlique.co.uk

Another range that is only available online, these products, suitable for even the most super-sensitive skins, include a variety for men's skin care. They are made from organically and biodynamically grown herbs from a dedicated farm in South Australia.

Neal's Yard Remedies
Tel.: 0845 262 3145
Website: www.nealsyardremedies.com

Produces a wide variety of products specially formulated for sensitive skins, which are available from over a hundred shops and stockists in the UK as well as online.

Weleda
Tel.: 0115 944 8222
Website: www.weleda.co.uk

Offers Dermatodoron Ointment (obtainable in pharmacies not health food shops) which is a licensed anthroposophic medicine for eczema, designed to be used in conjunction with other prescribed medicines.

Don't forget the High Street – **Boots** stores carry a range of cosmetics and toiletries suitable for sensitive skins in adults and children, as well as popular emollients such as E45 and Oilatum. Their 'Expert' Sensitive Skin range includes products for women, men and children. Your local store may have a skincare adviser accredited by the British Skin Foundation if you need more information about the products on sale. Some offer on-the-spot advice, others a free, pre-bookable consultation. Contact Customer Care on 0845 070 8090 for details.

Other products

Bio-Life Europe Ltd
1–3 Upper Grove End Farm Business Units
Henbrook Lane
Brailes
Oxon OX15 5BA
Tel.: 01608 686626
Website: www.bio-life.co.uk

Has a range of products to remove allergens, including Petal Cleanse, which is recommended for those whose eczema is affected by animal dander.

Green Building Store
Heath House Mill
Heath House Lane
Bolster Moor
West Yorkshire HD7 4JW
Tel.: 01484 461705
Website: www.greenbuildingstore.co.uk

Has a range of eco-friendly DIY products including paints (indoor and outdoor), wood preservatives and insulation, available to personal callers and through their mail-order and online store.

HealthGuard HealthCare Ltd
First Floor
707 High Road
North Finchley
London N12 0BT
Tel.: 020 8343 9911
Website: www.healthguardtm.com

Their HealthGuard Total Hygiene DM–1 Spray is specially formulated to remove dust-mite droppings which can cause eczema flare-ups and other allergic reactions.

Healthy Flooring Network
Tel.: 020 7481 9004
Website: www.healthyflooring.org

A source of advice on choosing appropriate flooring.

Outright Allergy Relief From Dogs/Cats is available by mail order from Bramton Company (01480 464550) or from pet stores.

Complementary therapies

Always ensure that any complementary practitioner you consult is a member of a reputable professional organization.

AcuMedic
101–105 Camden High Street
London NW1 7JN
Tel.: 020 7388 6704
Website: www.acumedic.com

AcuMedic Medical Centre and its sister company at the same address, Chinalife Body Clinic, have been established since 1972 for traditional Chinese medicine. There is also a branch in Bath (Tel.: 01225 483 393).

Avene Dermatological Spa
Tel.: 0033 (0) 467 23 41 87
Website: www.avenehydrotherapycenter.com

Spring water and other treatments have been used to treat skin conditions at this spa in south-western France for more than 200 years.

British Acupuncture Council
Tel.: 020 8735 0400
Website: www.acupuncture.org.uk

Can put you in touch with an accredited acupuncturist in your area.

British Autogenic Society
Tel.: 020 7391 8908
Website: www.autogenic-therapy.org.uk

Offers information about autogenic training, a simple self-help technique for stress management and relaxation.

British Homoeopathic Association
Tel.: 0870 444 3950
Website: www.trusthomeopathy.org

Provides information about local homoeopathic doctors.

British Society of Experimental and Clinical Hypnosis
Tel.: 01457 839363
Website: www.bsech.com

Can give information about hypnotherapy and details of local practitioners.

British Society of Medical and Dental Hypnosis
Tel.: 07000 560309
Website: www.bsmdh.org

Another group that offers information about hypnotherapy.

British Wheel of Yoga
Tel.: 01529 306851
Website: www.bwy.org.uk

Can give information about yoga teachers and classes in your area. Relaxing therapies such as yoga will not cure your eczema but are helpful in reducing stress.

National Institute of Medical Herbalists
Tel.: 01392 426022
Website: www.nimh.org.uk

Can refer you to a medical herbalist in your area.

Other sources of help

ChildLine
Tel.: 0800 1111
Website: www.childline.org.uk

An organization to help any child in danger or trouble, including those who are being bullied for any reason.

Kidscape
Tel.: 08451 205 204
Website: www.kidscape.org.uk

Provides information on bullying for children, parents, carers and teachers.

PetClub UK
Website: www.petclubuk.com

A website for pet-owners and potential pet-owners offering advice on choosing a pet which will not cause an allergic reaction. The site also gives hints on how to minimize allergic reaction to pets.

Sainsbury's/WellBeing 'Centre for Pregnancy Nutrition' Helpline: 08451 303646 (Weekdays, 10 a.m. to 4 p.m.)

Qualified dieticians can give advice on the latest findings concerning healthy eating for women who are pregnant or planning to become pregnant.

Further reading

Eckersley, Jill, *Coping with Childhood Allergies*, Sheldon Press, 2005.
Gazzola, Alex, *Living with Food Allergy*, Sheldon Press, 2006.
Gazzola, Alex, *Living with Food Intolerance*, Sheldon Press, 2005.

Index